D0467026

THE TRUTH ABOUT SEXUAL BEHAVIOR AND UNPLANNED PREGNANCY

THE TRUTH ABOUT SEXUAL BEHAVIOR AND UNPLANNED PREGNANCY

SECOND EDITION

Robert N. Golden, M.D.
University of Wisconsin–Madison
General Editor

Fred L. Peterson, Ph.D.
University of Texas–Austin
General Editor

Elissa Howard-Barr, Ph.D., and Stacey M. Barrineau
Principal Authors

William Kane, Ph.D.
University of New Mexico
Adviser to the First Edition

Mark J. Kittleson, Ph.D.
Southern Illinois University
Adviser to the First Edition

☑Facts On File
An imprint of Infobase Publishing

The Truth About Sexual Behavior and Unplanned Pregnancy, Second Edition

Facts On File, Inc.
An imprint of Infobase Publishing
132 West 31st Street
New York NY 10001

Library of Congress Cataloging-in-Publication Data

Howard-Barr, Elissa.
   The truth about sexual behavior and unplanned pregnancy / Robert N. Golden, general editor, Fred Peterson, general editor ; Elissa Howard-Barr and Stacey Barrineau, principal authors. − 2nd ed.
       p. cm. − (Truth about series)
   Rev. ed. of: The truth about sexual behavior and unplanned pregnancy / Mark J. Kittleson, general editor. c2005.
   Includes index.
   ISBN-13: 978-0-8160-7634-5 (hardcover : alk. paper)
   ISBN-10: 0-8160-7634-0 (hardcover : alk. paper) 1. Sex instruction for teenagers. 2. Teenagers−Sexual behavior. 3. Teenage pregnancy−Prevention. 4. Hygiene, Sexual. I. Golden, Robert N. II. Barrineau, Stacey. III. Truth about sexual behavior and unplanned pregnancy. IV. Title.
   HQ35.T78 2009
   613.9071'2−dc22

                                             2009008403

Facts On File books are available at special discounts when purchased in bulk quantities for businesses, associations, institutions, or sales promotions. Please call our Special Sales Department in New York at (212) 967-8800 or (800) 322-8755.

You can find Facts On File on the World Wide Web at http://www.factsonfile.com.

Text design by David Strelecky

Printed and bound in the United States of America

MP KC 10 9 8 7 6 5 4 3 2 1

This book is printed on acid-free paper.

CONTENTS

LIST OF ILLUSTRATIONS AND TABLES

PREFACE

The Truth About series—updated and expanded to include 20 volumes—seeks to identify the most pressing health issues and social challenges confronting our nation's youth. Adolescence is the period between the onset of puberty and the attainment of adult roles and responsibilities. Adolescence is also a time of storm, stress, and risk-taking for many young people. During adolescence, a person's health is influenced by biological, psychological, and social factors, all of which interact with one's environment—family, peers, school, and community. It is a time when teenagers experience profound changes.

With the latest available statistics and new insights that have emerged from ongoing research, the Truth About series seeks to help young people build a foundation of information as they face some of the challenges that will affect their health and well-being. These challenges include high-risk behaviors, such as alcohol, tobacco, and other drug use; sexual behaviors that can lead to adolescent pregnancy and sexually transmitted diseases (STDs), such as HIV/AIDS; mental health concerns, such as depression and suicide; learning disorders and disabilities, which are often associated with school failures and school drop outs; serious family problems, including domestic violence and abuse; and lifestyle factors, which increase adolescents' risk for noncommunicable diseases, such as diabetes and cardiovascular disease, among others.

Broader underlying factors also influence adolescent health. These include socioeconomic circumstances, such as poverty, available health care, and the political and social situations in which young people live. Although these factors can negatively affect adolescent health and well-being, as well as school performance, many of these negative health outcomes are preventable with the proper knowledge and information.

With prevention in mind, the writers and editors of each topical volume in the Truth About series have tried to provide cutting-edge information that is supported by research and scientific evidence. Vital facts are presented that inform youth about the challenges experienced during adolescence, while special features seek to dispel common myths and misconceptions. Some of the main topics explored include abuse, alcohol, death and dying, divorce, drugs, eating disorders, family life, fear and depression, rape, sexual behavior and unplanned pregnancy, smoking, and violence. All volumes discuss risk-taking behaviors and their consequences, healthy choices, prevention, available treatments, and where to get help.

In this new edition of the series, we also have added eight new titles in areas of increasing significance to today's youth. ADHD, or attention deficit/hyperactivity disorder, and learning disorders are diagnosed with increasing frequency, and many students have observed or know of classmates receiving treatment for these conditions, even if they have not themselves received this diagnosis. Gambling is gaining currency in our culture, as casinos open and expand in many parts of the country, and the Internet offers easy access for this addictive behavior. Another consequence of our increasingly "online" society, unfortunately, is the presence of online predators. Environmental hazards represent yet another danger, and it is important to provide unbiased information about this topic to our youth. Suicide, which for many years has been a "silent epidemic," is now gaining recognition as a major public health problem throughout a person's life span, including the teenage and young adult years. We now also offer an overview of illness and disease in a volume that includes the major conditions of particular interest and concern to youth. In addition to illness, however, it is essential to emphasize health and its promotion, and this is especially apparent in the volumes on physical fitness and stress management.

It is our intent that each book serve as an accessible, authoritative resource that young people can turn to for accurate and meaningful answers to their specific questions. The series can help them research particular problems and provide an up-to-date evidence base. It is also designed with parents, teachers, and counselors in mind so that they have a reliable resource that they can share with youth who seek their guidance.

Finally, we have tried to provide unbiased facts rather than subjective opinions. Our goal is to help elevate the health of the public with an emphasis on its most precious component—our youth. As young people face the challenges of an increasingly complex world, we as educators want them to be armed with the most powerful weapon available—knowledge.

Robert N. Golden, M.D.
Fred L. Peterson, Ph.D.
General Editors

HOW TO USE THIS BOOK

NOTE TO STUDENTS

Knowledge is power. By possessing knowledge you have the ability to make decisions, ask follow-up questions, or know where to go to obtain more information. In the world of health, that is power! That is the purpose of this book—to provide you the power you need to obtain unbiased, accurate information and *The Truth About Sexual Behavior and Unplanned Pregnancy*.

Topics in each volume of The Truth About are arranged in alphabetical order, from A to Z. Each of these entries defines its topic and explains in detail the particular issue. At the end of most entries are cross-references to related topics. A list of all topics by letter can be found in the table of contents or at the back of the book in the index.

How have these books been compiled? First, the publisher worked with me to identify some of the country's leading authorities on key issues in health education. These individuals were asked to identify some of the major concerns that young people have about such topics. The writers read the literature, spoke with health experts, and incorporated their own life and professional experiences to pull together the most up-to-date information on health issues, particularly those of interest to adolescents and of concern in Healthy People 2010.

Throughout the alphabetical entries, the reader will find sidebars that separate Fact from Fiction. There are Question-and-Answer boxes that attempt to address the most common questions that youth ask about sensitive topics. In addition, readers will find a special feature called "Teens Speak"—case studies of teens with personal stories related to the topic in hand.

This may be one of the most important books you will ever read. Please share it with your friends, families, teachers, and classmates. Remember, you possess the power to control your future. One way to affect your course is through the acquisition of knowledge. Good luck and keep healthy.

NOTE TO LIBRARIANS

This book, along with the rest of the Truth About series, serves as a wonderful resource for young researchers. It contains a variety of facts, case studies, and further readings that the reader can use to help answer questions, formulate new questions, or determine where to go to find more information. Even though the topics may be considered delicate by some, don't be afraid to ask patrons if they have questions. Feel free to direct them to the appropriate sources, but do not press them if you encounter reluctance. The best we can do as educators is to let young people know that we are there when they need us.

Mark J. Kittleson, Ph.D.
Adviser to the First Edition

RISK TAKING AND SEXUAL BEHAVIOR

Sexuality is a fundamental part of human development. The physical and emotional growth of people are in part shaped by sexuality and the ways in which society perceives it. There are many myths about sexual development and sexuality. It is important for young adults to be able to recognize facts and to dispel myths in order to create and maintain a healthy perception of sexuality.

NEW IN THE REVISED EDITION

In this new edition of *The Truth About Sexual Behavior and Unplanned Pregnancy*, all of the statistics have been revised to reflect the most recent information available. Updated graphs and charts include information and rates of abortion and sexually transmitted infections. There are updates about the cost of childcare—not just financial, but also the overall emotional toll that teens experience raising a child. There is additional information about physical and psychological changes during sexual development, as well as further description of the adverse reactions to alcohol and drugs, their effect on the brain, and how judgment is impaired.

Several sections have been added as "Teens Speak" for other teens to share their stories relating to experiences they have been through, from being born with birth defects to being the target of hate crimes. Also, with the unfortunate increase of online sex crimes and predators, additional statistics and information have been added regarding cyber sex.

There also are seven new sections that are of growing interest and importance, especially to young adults. An important component of stable growth and development is affection. "Affection, Appropriate" explains that when we are children, our parents show us affection by nurturing us and that warmth and affection contribute to secure relationships between people. The new section also defines what public display of affection is and how important it is that individuals involved in a relationship establish their own boundaries of what they feel is both appropriate and inappropriate regarding it.

"Birth Defects and Risk-Taking Behaviors" answers questions about how common birth defects really are and describes behaviors that pregnant women can avoid to lower the risk of birth defects. This section reveals that most birth defects happen during the first three months of pregnancy and that the cause of up to 70 percent of birth defects is still unknown. "Prenatal Care" parallels some of the topics discussed in "Birth Defects and Risk-Taking Behaviors" but better describes the importance of women getting proper health care when they find out they are pregnant and during their pregnancy.

What causes diabetes? Will my baby be affected if I have diabetes when I'm pregnant? Are there ways to maintain my health if I have diabetes and I'm pregnant? "Diabetes and Pregnancy" discusses the different types of diabetes, as well as focusing on gestational diabetes that can occur during pregnancy.

Additionally, "Hepatitis" covers the different types, causes, and prevention and treatments for this disease, while the section on "Pelvic Inflammatory Disease" uncovers myths and answers questions about what PID really is and how you can protect yourself.

The last addition is extremely significant for young people today. The dramatic increase of online crime and sexual predators is disturbing. "Sexual Predators" informs readers of the shocking trend that is escalating, noting that an estimated two out of every 10 girls and one out of every 10 boys are sexually abused by the age of 13.

UNDERSTANDING SEXUALITY

Being sexual is an essential part of being human. Throughout our lives, we make sexual choices based on our experiences, attitudes, values, and knowledge. With the addition of these new sections and the updates throughout this new edition, a more comprehensive picture of sexuality is painted for young people. Learning about sex can be scary, and some teens may be embarrassed to ask questions and seek answers. This text is designed to present answers to questions as clearly as possible and to be as user-friendly as possible.

Humans use their sexuality for **reproduction,** the process of creating offspring, but sexuality is about more than having a baby. Your gender—male or female—and your feelings about being male or female are part of your sexuality as well. Sexuality also includes your sexual orientation and your values and beliefs about life, love, and intimacy. Your sexuality influences how you feel about yourself and others and the way you experience the world.

SEXUALITY AND SOCIETY

Every group of people has rules or laws about sexual activities. In the United States, for example, it is a serious crime to force someone to engage in sexual behavior against his or her will. Americans believe that the decision to engage in sexual activity should be a matter of mutual choice. No one should be pressured or forced to have sex.

At the same time, Americans live in a sexually charged world. Sexuality is not only discussed but also on display wherever people gather—at the mall, on the playground, or at sports events. People of all ages are bombarded with messages about sex and sexual behavior on radio and TV, and in movies, magazines, and music.

Not surprisingly, many teens are confused about sexual behavior. They hear a lot about sex, but they receive few facts about the topics that concern them: What is normal? What is the difference between love and sex? How do I deal with peer pressure? How does someone get a sexually transmitted disease? Could I have one and not know it?

Those questions often stem from mixed messages regarding sexuality in the media. News programs and documentaries may provide useful information about the dangers of casual sex, even as entertainment programs show young, single people engaging in casual sex with no contraception, no consequences, and often no feelings for each other. A 2006 article in *Pediatrics & Adolescent Medicine* revealed that, among young adolescents, watching TV two or more hours per day and lack of parental regulation of TV programs being watched were each associated with increased risk of initiating sex within a year.

Every teen has to make important decisions about his or her sexuality—decisions that can have life-changing consequences. Potentially risky choices related to sexual behavior include unprotected sex, sex with multiple partners, or mixing alcohol and drugs with sex.

Learning to question images and stories in the media, finding reliable sources of information about sexuality, and developing supportive relationships with adults and other teens are essential to making good decisions.

PUBERTY

Everyone experiences **puberty,** but it doesn't happen to everyone at the same time. Puberty is the period during which a child's body becomes sexually mature and develops into an adult form. Generally, girls begin puberty earlier than boys. The bodies of some girls begin changing as early as eight years old. Other girls don't start developing until they are 14. Boys usually show signs of puberty between the ages of 10 and 12. Most often, puberty is complete by the time a teen has reached his or her 20th birthday.

For almost everyone, puberty is a time of rapid physical and emotional changes. It can be a tough time for many teens, particularly those who don't understand the changes that take place in their bodies. Some changes are the same for girls and boys. Both get taller and grow hair under their arms and around their sex organs. Both perspire more, too, mostly under the arms. The voices of both girls and boys deepen during puberty. The change is more sudden in boys and more gradual in girls.

Many of these changes are due to chemicals in the body known as **hormones.** Hormones target cells or organs by regulating such activities as growth and reproduction. Two of these hormones—estrogen in girls and testosterone in boys—guide children's development into women and men capable of having a baby.

Changes outside the body

Girls can see many of the changes that estrogen causes in their bodies. The first sign of puberty may be a white, sticky discharge from the vagina (female reproductive organ). It is normal and an indication of other changes to come. During puberty, a girl's breasts begin to develop and her hips get rounder.

Boys experience hormonal changes, too. A boy's **testes** (male reproductive organs that produce sperm) get bigger and hang lower. His **penis** (male sex organ) also grows larger and gets hard more often and unexpectedly.

Boys and girls usually develop a number of **secondary sex characteristics** during puberty. Secondary sex characteristics distinguish the sexes but are not directly related to reproduction. For example, boys may start growing beards after their voices change.

Hormonal changes can cause not only physical changes but also abrupt changes in mood. During puberty, many teens feel that they are on an emotional roller-coaster ride.

Changes inside the body

Important changes also take place inside the body. During puberty, girls experience **menstruation** for the first time. Menstruation is the loss of blood and tissue lining the **uterus** that happens each month when a woman does not become pregnant. The uterus is the hollow organ in a female's body in which a baby develops. As girls mature, the eggs in their ovaries begin to ripen. Eggs are the female reproductive cells.

Boys experience their first **nocturnal emission,** or wet dream, meaning they have begun producing **sperm,** male reproductive cells. They can now cause pregnancy.

Pregnancy can occur if a single sperm joins with an egg. So, a female can get pregnant if a male inserts his penis in or near her vagina. A teen's reproductive system matures faster than he or she does, which is why girls can get pregnant and boys can cause pregnancy before they are fully grown.

DATING AND RELATIONSHIPS

Teens often begin to date during puberty. Dating provides young people with an opportunity to get to know another person in a romantic way and enjoy one another's company. Exactly when a teen begins to date varies greatly. Some teens are interested in dating earlier than others. Families also have rules that may affect when a teen is allowed to go out on a date.

Experts suggest that teens should not date just because their friends are dating. They should start a dating relationship because they have met someone they care about and want to know better.

A healthy dating relationship has many of the characteristics of a healthy friendship. Both require good communication skills, honesty, and mutual respect. In a healthy relationship, neither partner pressures the other to do something against his or her will. Teens who are dating should respect their partner's right to say no to anything that makes him or her feel uncomfortable. By talking about how they feel about things, teens may avoid getting into situations where they feel pressured into making a decision on the spot about something important.

The Center for Young Women's Health at Children's Hospital in Boston offers the following tips for starting a healthy and safe dating relationship:

- Get to know a person by talking on the phone or at school before you go out for the first time.
- On the first few dates, go out with a group of friends to a public place.
- Plan fun activities like going to the movies, a picnic, a ball game, or a party.
- Be sure the other person knows what you feel comfortable doing and when you're expected home by your parent(s) or guardian.
- Tell at least one friend and especially your parent(s) where you are going, who you will be with, and how to reach you.

SEXUAL ABUSE

Safety is an important issue in dating today. According to recent studies, it is extremely likely that you or someone you know has experienced abuse in a dating relationship. The abuse may be physical, psychological, or emotional as well as sexual. Psychological and emotional abuse may include swearing at or insulting a partner, embarrassing him or her, or making threats. Physical abuse includes hitting, shoving, or slapping. Sexual abuse refers to forced or unwanted sexual activity or rape.

According to the National Youth Violence Prevention Resource Center, it is difficult to get accurate information about the extent of violence related to dating. Teens rarely report abusive relationships and the few studies that ask about them do so in different ways. Some ask only about sexual abuse, while others include questions about emotional and psychological abuse.

The 2007 Youth Risk Behavior Surveillance System (YRBSS) survey by the Centers for Disease Control and Prevention (CDC) found that 8.8 percent of girls and 11 percent of boys had been hit, slapped, or physically harmed by a boyfriend or girlfriend in the previous year. In grades 9–12, 11.3 percent of girls and 4.5 percent of boys also reported that they had been forced to have sexual intercourse against their will.

Any forced sexual activity is considered a **sexual assault**. According to the Department of Justice (DOJ), an estimated 191,670 assaults were reported in the United States in 2005. According to the Florida Council against Sexual Violence, rape is the most underreported crime in America, so it is difficult to know how many lives are affected by sexual violence. The Bureau of Justice Statistics estimates that only 41.1 percent of victims report the crime to law enforcement. One out of every 10 adult women has been the victim of forcible rape, which is more than 12 million women in America.

In the United States, one in six women and one in 33 men reported experiencing an attempted or completed rape at some time in their lives. Additionally, 75.8 percent of rape or sexual assault victims knew their offenders, according to the Department of Justice in 2005. Not all sexual assaults involve brute force. Some assailants use drugs or alcohol to sexually assault another person. Common date rape drugs include alcohol, Rohypnol, and GHB. All of these drugs are **depressants**—drugs that slow the central nervous system, including breathing. Rohypnol and GHB can cause a person to black out for up to 12 hours and not remember anything that happened.

People who commit sexual assaults are punished if the assault is reported and they are found guilty. When someone uses a drug, such as Rohypnol or GHB, they may face serious jail time and a high fine. These drugs are against the law, and giving them to someone without their consent is illegal.

TEENS AND SEXUALITY

The YRBSS (administered every other year by the CDC) provides valuable information about teens and their relationships. According to the 2007 survey, about 47.8 percent of all teens in the United States have had sex before they graduated from high school. About 14.9 percent have had four or more partners. Teens today have sex for a variety of reasons. Some are curious. Others want to please their partner or feel their partner will only stay with them if they have sex.

Other teens realize that they are not ready to have sex. Some want to wait until they are more mature, while others prefer to wait until they are married. Still others do not have sex because they are afraid of pregnancy or getting a sexually transmitted disease (STD).

Teens and contraceptives

Teens who decide to have sex should use a **contraceptive** (a device to prevent an unwanted pregnancy). According to the CDC's 2007 YRBSS survey, 77 percent of American teens use contraceptives when they have sex. Any time couples have unprotected sex, they risk a pregnancy. They also risk getting an STD. Many times when teens have sex, drugs and alcohol are involved. When someone is drunk or high, he or she is less likely to use a contraceptive than if he or she were sober and thinking clearly.

Reliable contraceptives include **condoms** and the **birth control pill.** A condom, made of thin rubberlike material called latex, covers the penis during sexual intercourse or oral sex. A condom protects against both pregnancy and STDs and can be purchased at a drug store without a prescription. The birth control pill is a hormonal method of birth control that prevents **ovulation,** the release of an egg from a female's ovary. The pill protects only against pregnancy.

Other methods of contraception may not be as reliable. These include **withdrawal,** or pulling out, and the **rhythm method,** avoiding intercourse around the time of ovulation. Withdrawal is risky because a male cannot always determine when he will ejaculate. It requires a lot of control, which can be difficult for young males. The rhythm method is unreliable because a woman, especially in her teen years, may have difficulty determining exactly when she is ovulating. Also, sperm can live in a woman's body for up to three days, so there is about a week within each month when a woman should avoid intercourse.

Teens and sexually transmitted diseases

Of all contraceptives available, the condom is the only one that reduces the risk of contracting an STD. According to the CDC in 2008, one in four sexually active teenage girls has an STD. The CDC also estimates that approximately 19 million new STD infections occur each year, almost half of them among young people ages 15–24 years old. Someone with a viral STD could be contagious even without symptoms. Viral STDs, which include HIV, herpes, and genital warts, do not go away. A person with a viral STD is likely to have it for life.

Bacterial STDs can be treated with antibiotics if a person knows he or she has one. Unfortunately, most STDs have no symptoms or symptoms that are very mild, increasing the chances that one may be unaware that he or she has an STD. For example, males and females with chlamydia, a bacterial STD, do not have symptoms 80 percent of the time, which is why it is so important to get tested.

Most doctors will test for STDs if asked and most county or state health departments provide free or very inexpensive STD testing. Planned Parenthood and local health clinics offer STD testing as well. Testing is important for anyone who has been **raped** (forced to have intercourse against his or her will).

Teen pregnancy, childbirth, and parenting

According to the National Campaign to Prevent Teenage Pregnancy, between 1991 and 2005, the U.S. birthrate for teens aged 15–19 declined 35 percent to 40.4 births per 1,000 teen girls, after reaching its highest point in two decades in 1991 (61.8 births per 1,000 teen girls aged 15–19). Between 2005 and 2006, preliminary data suggest that rates have risen approximately 3 percent. While the overall trend toward decrease is encouraging, the U.S. teen birthrate remains notably higher than the rates in other industrialized countries. According to Advocates for Youth, U.S. teens account for about 7 percent of all teenage births occurring in all developed countries. The United States's teen birth rate is more than four times higher than Germany's, four and a half times higher than France's, and almost nine times higher than that of the Netherlands. Each year, about one million teens in the United States become pregnant. They have several options. They can have the baby and raise it, give the child up for adoption, or have an abortion.

If a woman decides to have her baby, she will go through pregnancy. During pregnancy, prenatal care is essential for both the woman and her baby. Regular checkups, proper nutrition, and avoiding drugs and alcohol help to ensure the health of the developing fetus as well as the expectant mother. Everything a woman eats, drinks, or injects into her body goes directly to the baby. No drug or alcohol is safe. Doctors do not recommend that a woman take even a cold tablet or an aspirin during pregnancy.

Pregnancy is usually divided into three stages.

The first trimester, or first three months of pregnancy, is characterized by rapid growth of the **fetus** (the developing child from the second month of pregnancy until birth). The heartbeat begins on day 21 and all organs begin to function by month three. The fetus, which is now about three inches long, sleeps, wakes, and exercises muscles.

During the second trimester, the next three months, the fetus continues to grow and develop. By the sixth month, the fetus is 10–12 inches long and weighs about one pound. By then, the fetus can hear and open his or her eyes. He or she has fingernails, eyebrows, eyelashes, and possibly hair.

During the last three months, or the third trimester, the fetus gains weight rapidly and grows from about 11 to 13 inches in the seventh month to 19 or 20 inches by the ninth month.

Childbirth is also characterized by three stages. The first stage, lasting from two to 12 hours on average, begins with contractions, the woman's water breaking, or the dilation, or expanding, of the **cervix.** The cervix is the small opening to the uterus. The cervix must expand to allow the fetus to pass through. The term *water breaking* is commonly used to describe the rupture of the **amniotic sac,** a thin protective membrane filled with fluid that protects the developing fetus. The woman may feel this fluid leaving her body.

The second stage, which lasts from 30 minutes to two hours, involves pushing, or actively bearing down to help squeeze or push the baby out. Pain medications may be used to lessen a woman's discomfort during this time.

Finally, when the baby is out, the birth of the **placenta** occurs. It is the third stage of childbirth. The placenta is the organ through which the fetus received nourishment.

Becoming a parent during one's teen years is a challenge. Raising a baby is a full-time job that usually requires overtime. Childrearing may affect one's ability to attend school, hold a job, or even spend time with friends. The best way to prevent an unwanted pregnancy is to not have sex or to always use a contraceptive during sex.

SEXUAL EXPRESSION

Individuals express their sexuality in many different ways. Sexual expression is more than sexual intercourse. It also includes kissing, hugging, and touching. Some individuals choose **celibacy.** They abstain from sexual behavior for personal or religious reasons. Other people practice **masturbation,** the stimulation of the genitals with hands. Some choose this form of sexual expression to remain a virgin or avoid an unwanted pregnancy or STDs.

Oral sex is another way to express sexuality. One partner puts his or her mouth or tongue on the genitals of his or her partner. Although oral sex cannot result in pregnancy, it can put someone at risk for contracting an STD.

Intercourse, either vaginal or anal, involves penetration of the penis into the vagina or anus. Vaginal intercourse may result in an unwanted pregnancy and/or an STD. Using a condom every time is important to avoid both risks. Also, vaginal intercourse is not recommended immediately after anal intercourse. Bacteria from the anus can cause a serious infection in the vagina.

Some people express their sexuality in **autoerotic behavior,** such as through fantasies or erotic dreams. These are normal mental experiences that many teens experience. Other variations of sexual expressions, including **fetishes** and **exhibitionism,** may be dangerous to others and therefore illegal. A fetish is an infatuation with an object or body part that causes sexual arousal. Exhibitionism is the illegal exposure of one's genitals to someone without his or her consent. Exhibitionists are also called flashers.

Sexual orientation

A person's sexual orientation describes his or her enduring attraction to another person. Those who are attracted to a member of the opposite sex are **heterosexual.** Those who are attracted to a member of the same sex are **homosexual.** People who are attracted to members of both the same and opposite sex are **bisexual.** A person cannot choose his or her sexual orientation.

Although American society is becoming more accepting of homosexuals, **homophobia** still exists. Homophobia is an intense, irrational fear and hatred of homosexuals. People with severe homophobia may commit crimes against homosexuals and believe they are justified in harming them. It is never right to judge or harm anyone due to their sexual orientation.

Community services

Many communities provide a variety of services for teens related to sexuality—including rape crisis centers, family planning clinics, adoption agencies, shelters, and public health departments. Some offer prenatal care, STD screening and treatment, counseling, and birth control. People can locate these services in their own community by looking in the Yellow Pages, asking an adult, or searching on the Internet.

Sexuality is all around us—in the media, in school, and at home. It can be negative or positive. Knowing the facts, knowing oneself, and, most important, knowing about protection is critical. By being open about sexuality and talking about the issues, people will better know how to protect themselves and where to go for help if needed.

RISKY BUSINESS SELF-TESTS

Test 1: Do you have a realistic attitude about love?

Love does not mean the same thing to everyone. What does it mean to you? Keep a record of your answers to the following statements on a piece of paper.

	Strongly Agree	Somewhat Agree	Strongly Disagree
1. Research should not be done on love. Love should remain mysterious.	3	2	1
2. Love is the most important thing in my life.	3	2	1
3. My life is very unhappy when I am not in love.	3	2	1
4. I am able to function well without someone to love.	1	2	3
5. Love is a fantasy that is popular with teenage girls.	1	2	3
6. Each of us has a "one and only" out there.	3	2	1
7. Once you find your "one and only," you will never become attracted to anyone else.	3	2	1
8. If you love someone too much, you will get hurt.	1	2	3
9. I am able to function well without someone loving me.	1	2	3

10. The smartest people don't get hung up on another person.	1	2	3
11. You can tell when you first meet someone whether you are going to love that person.	3	2	1
12. The best relationships have a basis more important than love.	1	2	3
13. If you love someone enough, any problem in the relationship can be overcome.	3	2	1
14. If I had to choose between living in poverty or living without love, I would choose poverty.	3	2	1
15. As soon as someone thinks you love him or her, that person will take advantage of you.	1	2	3
16. You're a fool if you fall in love with someone who has no money.	1	2	3

Total points: _____

Interpretations:

40–48 points: You have very romantic ideas about love. You might put too much emphasis on love as the only basis for a partnership, while ignoring other important considerations.

24–39 points: You have a realistic idea about love. Although love is important to you, you also are aware of the many other aspects of a smoothly functioning partnership.

16–23 points: You appear to be cynical about love. Maybe you were hurt before or came from a family where romance was not emphasized. Your attitudes might insulate you from getting hurt again, but they could also prevent you from enjoying the benefits of a loving relationship.

Source: Byer, Curtis O., Louis W. Shainberg, and Grace Galliano. *Dimensions of Human Sexuality.* 6th ed. Boston: McGraw-Hill, 2001.

Test 2: Talking to your parent(s) or guardian

One of the most valuable resources teens have is their parent(s) or guardian. Think about your answers to the following questions. Next, ask a parent or guardian to do the same. Then, compare your responses with his or hers.

1. What characteristics do you feel are necessary to have/develop a healthy relationship and why?

2. How should teenagers show affection to a significant person (boy-friend/girlfriend) in their life?

3. How do you feel about teenagers who choose to be sexually active prior to marriage?

4. What can parent(s) do to help their child(ren) avoid an unwanted pregnancy, sexually transmitted disease, or heartache from an unhealthy relationship?

5. How is dating today different compared to when your parent(s) were teenagers?

6. What did I learn about talking to my parent(s) about healthy relationships?

7. What did I learn about taking to my son/daughter about healthy relationships?

Source: Tackman, Deborah. *Outrageous Teaching Techniques in Health Education.* Eau Claire, Wis.: Deborah Tackman, 2006.

A TO Z ENTRIES

■ ABORTION

The ending of a pregnancy before the developing baby is able to survive. Abortions occur in a variety of ways. Some abortions are the result of natural causes. Others are intentional acts.

In 2005, 1.21 million abortions were performed, down from 3.1 million in 2000. According to the Guttmacher Institute, a group that researches issues related to health and public education, more than one-half of the women who decide to have an abortion are in their twenties. Approximately 20 percent are under age 19. Therefore, teens make up about one in five of all abortions. Over one-half of all abortions are performed on women who used contraception incorrectly or used a method that failed.

TYPES OF ABORTION

There are two types of abortions—**spontaneous abortions** and **elective abortions.** Spontaneous abortions refer to termination of pregnancies due to natural causes at less than 20 weeks into a pregnancy. Elective abortions mean choosing to end a pregnancy before the developing baby can survive.

Experts say that up to 50 percent of all fertilized eggs die and are aborted spontaneously, usually before the woman knows she is pregnant. According to Planned Parenthood, for every 10 pregnancies, one to two end in miscarriage. Miscarriage is most likely to happen early in pregnancy—in fact, eight out of 10 miscarriages happen in the first three months of pregnancy.

The cause of most spontaneous abortions, or **miscarriages,** is fetal death due to abnormalities, usually unrelated to the mother. Other possible causes for a spontaneous abortion include infections, physical problems the mother may have, hormonal problems, immune responses, and diseases in the mother. The risk for spontaneous abortion is higher in women over the age of 35 and women with a history of three or more prior spontaneous abortions.

A miscarriage may also be caused by a damaged **cervix** (the opening to the uterus); diabetes; cocaine use; or an abnormal uterus. A healthy pregnant woman cannot cause a miscarriage by jumping, vigorously exercising, or engaging in intercourse.

When a spontaneous abortion occurs, hormone levels drop and the lining of the **uterus** (the hollow organ located in the lower abdomen that houses a developing baby) begins to shed. The fetus separates from the uterus and passes out of the body. A woman who is having a miscarriage will feel severe cramps and begin to bleed. Seeing a doctor is important after a miscarriage to determine if there are other complications.

Q & A

Question: Can a woman still have a healthy pregnancy after a miscarriage?

Answer: Many women do. Having a miscarriage usually does not endanger future pregnancies. Most women can still get pregnant again and have a healthy baby. Some women may even have two or three miscarriages before carrying a baby to term. A miscarriage can be a very difficult experience. Some couples may experience guilt, anger, and grief. Most couples need time to grieve before they are willing to consider trying to get pregnant again.

An elective abortion occurs when a woman chooses to end her pregnancy. Nine in 10 abortions occur within the first 12 weeks of pregnancy. Physicians perform most abortion procedures. Between five and 13 weeks after the last menstrual period, they may do **suction curettage,** a procedure in which the doctor dilates the cervix and inserts a small plastic tube attached to a small vacuum into the uterus. The fetal tissue, placenta, and built-up uterine lining is then drawn, or suctioned, out. The procedure takes about 10 minutes at a clinic or hospital. Patients generally receive **anesthesia,** drugs given before and during surgery for relief of pain and sensation.

Dilation and evacuation (D and E) is the most common technique for ending a pregnancy between weeks 13 and 21. This procedure involves suction equipment, special forceps, and a **curette** (a metal instrument to scrape the uterine walls). Anesthesia is usually required. During this procedure, the cervix is dilated wider than it is during a suction curettage, and the uterus is scraped after the suctioning.

Risks involved with suction curettage and D and E include uterine infection, bleeding, or incomplete removal of the uterine contents. Most doctors require a follow-up visit to ensure there were no complications.

Prostaglandin induction is performed between 14 and 26 weeks. As of 2007, 36 states prohibit some abortions after a certain point in pregnancy. This type of abortion is rare and accounted for less than 1 percent of all abortions in 2003, according to the Guttmacher Institute. Prostaglandin induction, which is sometimes referred to as a "late term abortion," is usually performed only if the expectant mother's life is at risk or the fetus is not developing properly. During this procedure, the woman is given hormones that cause uterine contractions. A suppository may be placed in the vagina or a needle inserted into the amniotic sac (a thin-walled membrane that surrounds the fetus during pregnancy) through the abdominal wall to cause severe cramps and, within 24 hours, the expulsion of the fetus from the vagina.

A drug to induce abortion, RU-486, became available in the United States in 2000. RU-486 may eventually become the most common procedure for abortions within the first seven weeks of pregnancy. The drug blocks the hormone progesterone. Without this hormone, the cervix softens, the lining of the uterus breaks down, and bleeding begins. A few days later the woman takes the drug misoprostal, which causes the uterus to contract and expel the embryonic sac, which is about the size of a grape. This form of abortion has no side effects for some women but may cause cramping, headaches, nausea, or vomiting for others.

Fact Or Fiction?

The morning after pill is different from RU-486.

The Facts: The morning-after pill, known as **emergency contraception** (EC), is different from RU-486, the abortion pill. EC uses hormones to prevent fertilization or stop a fertilized egg from implanting in the uterus. It will not terminate an established pregnancy nor will it cause any harm to a developing fetus. Therefore, EC is not an abortion pill but a pill to prevent pregnancy after intercourse. A woman takes two pills within 72 hours of having unprotected sex. Information about EC is available on the Planned Parenthood Web site at http://www.plannedparenthood.org. EC is not meant for use as birth control.

THE CONTROVERSY OVER ABORTION

Until 1973, abortions were illegal in most states within the United States. In January of that year, the U.S. Supreme Court ruled in the case of *Roe v. Wade* that a woman has the right to decide whether to end or continue her pregnancy. A person's right to privacy includes a woman's decision, in consultation with her physician, to terminate her pregnancy, however, it is not an unlimited right.

The Court ruled that a woman has the right to choose until her fetus is viable—that is, until the fetus can survive outside the woman's body. At that time, a state may ban an abortion that is not necessary to preserve a woman's life or health.

As a result of *Roe v. Wade*, abortions are legal in every state. However, state laws regulating abortion vary greatly. Currently every state allows abortion during the first trimester. During the second trimester, some states either do not allow abortions or place restrictions on them. Abortions are illegal in all states during the third trimester unless the mother's life is at risk or the developing fetus has severe abnormalities.

The Court's ruling is controversial among the population. Some groups have hailed the decision, noting that before abortions were legal, some women induced an abortion with pills, herbs, or laxatives or by inserting sharp objects like a metal coat hanger through the vagina into the uterus. Others sought "back alley" abortions—abortions performed illegally and often under unsafe conditions. According to the Guttmacher Institute, there are an estimated 19 million unsafe abortions worldwide each year, most in low-income countries. About 5.2 million of these women are hospitalized for serious complications, while an unknown but possibly equal number of women suffer similarly serious complications but cannot obtain treatment. As a result, around 68,000 women die each year, making unsafe abortion a significant cause of maternal mortality.

Some states require **parental consent**—approval from at least one parent prior to permitting an abortion on a female under the age of 18. The Planned Parenthood Web site, www.plannedparenthood.org, details laws regarding abortion in each state.

TAKING SIDES

Some people consider themselves to be **pro-life** or **pro-choice**. Pro-life advocates believe that abortion should be illegal in all situations, even in the case of rape or incest or when the mother's life is at risk. Those who are pro-choice believe that abortion should be legal in all situations. They feel that the decision to have an abortion should be the woman's choice. Most people fall somewhere in between these views. They favor abortion in some situations and oppose it in others, although they may still align themselves with one side or the other.

Number of Legal Abortions Performed in the United States, 1973–2003

Year	Number of Abortions
1973	615,831
1983	1,268,987
1993	1,330,414
2003	848,163

Source: The Centers for Disease Control and Prevention, 2004.

Pro-life

The term **antiabortion activist** describes a person who actively works to outlaw all abortion by speaking publicly against the procedure. Some activists protest outside clinics where abortions are performed. Others harass people who enter the clinics by calling them names and posting antiabortion literature on their cars.

Pro-life extremists are a small group within the pro-life movement who strongly favor abolishing all abortions. They express their feelings about abortion by intimidating and sometimes hurting or even killing those who seek abortions or provide them.

Some extremists block abortion clinic entrances and harass patients and staff. Others have burned or bombed abortion clinics; the first such attack occurred in 1978. A few have murdered doctors who perform abortions. These people believe the deaths are justified to save unborn babies.

Extremists have also attacked the newly approved RU-486 abortion pill. Several have threatened doctors who prescribe it, stating they will be "hunted down." Just because someone doesn't agree with the use of RU-486 or other forms of abortion does not mean they have the right to hurt people to get their point across.

Extremists also make the false claim that many abortions occur during the latter stages of pregnancy. In reality, only about 1 percent of all abortions occur after 20 weeks of pregnancy, according to the Guttmacher Institute. Opponents call these abortions *partial birth abortions*. This term is not a medically recognized term. The

Violence and Disruption against Abortion Providers

	Murders, attempted murders	Bombing, arson, attempted bombing or arson	Invasion, assault and battery, vandalism, trespassing, death threats, burglary, stalking	Hate mail, harassing phone calls, bomb threats	Arrests made at blockades	Number of blockades	Number of picketing incidents
1992	0	32	221	1,481	2,580	83	2,898
1993	2	20	430	650	1,236	66	2,279
1994	12	15	143	395	217	25	1,407
1995	1	16	142	296	54	5	1,356
1996	1	9	102	618	65	7	3,932
1997	2	16	205	2,908	29	25	7,518
1998	3	10	127	946	16	2	8,402
1999	0	10	326	1,685	5	3	8,727
2000	1	5	209	1,031	0	4	8,478
2001	0	5	790	435	0	2	9,969
2002	0	1	265	302	0	4	10,241
2003	0	3	140	331	0	10	11,244
2004	0	3	145	466	0	34	11,640
2005	0	8	753	526	0	4	13,415
2006	0	4	469	555	0	13	13,505
2007	0	4	244	528	3	7	11,113
2008	0	1	48	90	0	1	2,648

Source: The National Abortion Federation, 2008.

correct term is *late term abortion*. These abortions are only done to save the life of the woman or to terminate a fetus with severe fetal abnormalities.

Pro-choice

People who consider themselves pro-choice believe that the decision to have an abortion should be the woman's choice. Because she is the one who carries the fetus for nine months and goes through childbirth, she has the right to decide whether to continue the pregnancy or end it. Although some people who are pro-choice believe that abortion is morally wrong, they also feel that the decision to have one belongs solely to the woman.

ABORTION AS A SUBSTITUTE FOR CONTRACEPTION

Although abortion remains legal, it is not an acceptable form of contraception. Deciding whether to have an abortion is a major decision—one that can be emotionally difficult, even painful. Some women later regret the choice they made. Considering all of the options and thinking them through is important to making the right decision for the woman involved. By using contraceptives correctly and consistently, more people can avoid having to make this difficult decision.

Abortion is a sensitive topic about which people hold strong opinions. Ultimately it is up to each woman to decide if abortion is right for her. The best way for couples to prevent an unwanted pregnancy is to use contraceptives every time they have sex, thus reducing the risk of having to make a decision regarding abortion.

TEENS SPEAK

I Had an Abortion Six Weeks Ago

I think I made the right choice, but sometimes I wish I had decided to keep the baby. When I found out I was pregnant, I was scared. Dave and I were not ready to get married. I wasn't even sure I wanted to see him any more. The first thing that popped into my head was to not have the baby.

Then I told Dave about the baby. He and his whole family wanted me to have it. My mother was furious. She didn't want me to have a baby. So, I was torn between his family and mine.

Now that I had the abortion, his family doesn't want to talk to me anymore. But you know what—I don't care.

In the long run, I feel I made the right choice. I really want to graduate and I don't see how I could take care of a baby and stay in school. My best friend had a baby last year. She stayed in school for a while, but in the end she dropped out. She couldn't handle it, and I don't think I could either.

See also: Contraceptives Involving Risk; Sex and the Law

FURTHER READING

The Guttmacher Institute. "Fact Sheet: An Overview of Abortion in the U.S." Available online. URL: http://www.guttmacher.org/media/presskits/2005/06/28/abortionoverview.html.

National Abortion and Reproductive Rights Action League Foundation. *Who Decides? A State-by-State Review of Abortion and Reproductive Rights.* Washington, D.C.: NARAL Foundation, 2003.

Pertman, Adam. *Adoption Nation: How the Adoption Revolution Is Transforming America.* New York: Basic Books, 2001.

ABSTINENCE
See: Contraceptives: Practices Proven Safe

AFFECTION, APPROPRIATE
A form or type of communication between people, where each individual gives and receives a certain amount of contact. We all need affection. Human beings are socially connected, and we are designed to show and receive affection. Affection has long been considered to be among the most basic and necessary human needs. The expression of affection is one of the primary communication methods humans use to develop and maintain quality relationships. It contributes to physical health, mental well-being, and academic performance. It also alleviates loneliness and depression. Often, it is through one's

expression of affection for another that a relationship is formed or transformed; People often remember the first hug, the first kiss, or the first time the words "I love you" were spoken. Affection is truly a central part of many social and personal relationships.

Affection is something exchanged between people, something that one gives and one receives. From infancy onward, it is the way we show others in our lives how important they are to us. Affection is the way humans express positive emotions. Holding hands, giving a hug or kiss, or simply smiling are all examples of affection.

WHY IS AFFECTION IMPORTANT?

Affection is a building block of human social development and life skills. From early childhood, it is crucial to give and receive affection. Beginning when we are children, our parents show us affection by nurturing us. Warmth and affection contribute to secure relationships between people. We can have a need for affection with just about anyone or anything. You feel affection for a family pet or for your parents. You also feel affection toward friends and romantic interests. What is so unique about our need for affection is that it can have varying degrees of intensity, depending on each of your specific relationships.

Parents are usually physically affectionate to children when they are young, but as these same children become teens, the children often balk at displays of affection from their parents, especially in public. Physical affection is important. Teens need their parents to continue being affectionate toward them because that allows respect and boundaries to form.

When we are comfortable enough to express ourselves through affection, we learn how to develop and maintain healthy relationships. Affection allows others to learn self-expression and to build self-esteem. Affection contributes to one's overall physical and mental well-being by making us feel safe and wanted. Affection is also a fundamental principal in **friendship** and love.

Fact Or Fiction?

Affectionate people tend to feel less stress and experience better mental health.

The Facts: According to Professor Kory Floyd's recent book, *Communicating Affection,* affection has distinct physical effects for both the receiver and the giver. Being affectionate is good for you; it is a low-cost way to reduce stress. Furthermore, there are direct associations between being an affectionate person and having a lower risk of depression and stress. Such associations include feeling acceptance from others, developing self-esteem, and returning affection to others.

APPROPRIATE AFFECTION

The desire for physical contact is basic human **nature**. However, there are times when affection can be deemed appropriate or inappropriate. It is important that the individuals involved in a relationship establish their own boundaries of what they feel is appropriate and not appropriate in terms of affection. It is up to each individual to establish the level at which he or she feels most comfortable in expressing affection toward others.

Public display of affection

Another facet of appropriate and inappropriate affection relates to displays of affection in public, typically referred to as **public display of affection (PDA)**. PDA can be holding hands or getting a peck on the cheek, but it could also be a passionate kiss. Many schools have created standards and rules for what is appropriate when it comes to showing affection in public. The schools have designed these standards and rules because they feel that showing PDA is a distraction and that it allows for a shift of focus away from the educational process. Many feel that it is ultimately up to the individuals involved in the relationship to determine their boundaries with what they feel comfortable expressing in public, school or otherwise.

TEENS SPEAK

New Rules at School

I hadn't ever really thought about whether I should kiss my boyfriend in public or not. I mean, we're dating, right? That's what people do. No one ever seemed to care. And lots of other kids do it. You see them at their lockers, or sitting on the stairs between classes. Everyone once in a while someone might say, "Get a room." But I just think they're jealous. At least, I figured that's all it was. But then last year the school passed a new rule banning PDA and made a huge deal out of everything.

I could see, maybe, banning kissing. I mean, sometimes it makes me uncomfortable watching people kiss at restaurants and things, so I guess the same thing could be true in the hall. But this new rule goes way beyond that. Derrick and I can't even hold hands! And last week my best friend Caroline got in trouble for running up to a bunch of her friends and giving them hugs! The teacher who saw her gave her detention for breaking the No PDA rule.

It got people upset. Her parents called the principal, and it even made it into the local newspaper. I think the school was afraid that kissing might lead to other things. But hugging your friends? They need to stop taking things so seriously.

The need for affection varies across cultural and geographical lines. In Europe, greeting someone by kissing each cheek is considered normal, while Americans like to greet each other with a handshake or a hug. Still the ultimate goal of fulfilling the need for affection is the same across all lines and cultural barriers—singling someone out and making that person feel special at a particular moment.

EMOTION AND AFFECTION

Giving and receiving affection means understanding our own emotions as well. The difference between emotion and affection is that an emotion is something internally felt, while affection is an expression of that internal feeling. Showing affection can be difficult for certain people because it may be regarded as a sign of weakness. Perhaps a person has trouble physically displaying emotions. Giving affection can be just as important as receiving it and can offer a person a sense of emotional release and fulfillment.

Affection can be expressed through verbal and nonverbal communication. The majority of all communication is nonverbal, and that includes gestures that show affection. We send messages through our eye contact, touch, and proximity to one another. If someone we're talking to touches our hand or arm, looks into our eyes, and leans toward us when we talk, we get the message that the person is interested in us and cares. There are also the obvious verbal expressions such as "I love you" that show our affection toward others as well. These are all gestures of affection that show our emotions. Fulfilling the need for affection requires us to let people into our minds and our hearts.

TEENS SPEAK

He Finally Said It

My name's Lisa, and I've been seeing Jason for like a year now. We started going out sophomore year. It's actually been really great. He's a lot of fun, always goofing around and making me laugh. We see movies together, do homework together, and when one of us has the money, sometimes we go out for dinner. I care about him a lot. But sometimes I wonder if he feels the same way.

I'd wanted to tell him that I love him for months. I kept thinking about it, trying to plan the right moment. But what if he didn't feel that way about me? I mean, what if I said it and he said, like, "That's nice," or "Cool"?

I came close a few times to just saying it anyway. But then we went to the park to take a walk and look at the pond. It didn't seem like a special day or anything. I could sense Jason kind of staring at me, though. Acting antsy. He took my hand, and I asked him if he was okay. Then he said he loved me.

It was what I'd been waiting to hear, but now that he'd said it, I couldn't help but wonder why. Did he want something? Was he going to ask me to sleep with him? I heard one of his friends telling him that we should have done it already. Was that why he said it?

It was nothing like the moment I'd planned. And I got so flustered that I didn't tell him I loved him back. His face turned red and he said we should head back home. I haven't seen him for a couple of days, and I don't know what to do now. I think I upset him, but I don't know what to say to make it better.

See also: Dating; Relationships and Responsibilities.

FURTHER READING
Bloom, Allison. "Is PDA Okay?" Teen Wire, 2005. Available online. URL: http://www.teenwire.com/infocus/2005/if-20050107p340-PDA.php. Accessed January 12, 2009.

■ BASICS OF GENDER IDENTITY, THE
A subjective but persistent sense of oneself as male or female. Unlike sexual identity, which refers to one's attraction to people of the same or the opposite sex, gender identity refers to an individual's personal sense of being male or female. Gender identity is more than simply looking like a female or male. Biological processes that begin after **conception**, the fusion of the egg and sperm, and cultural influences during early childhood both play a role.

UNDERSTANDING SEXUALITY
Sexuality encompasses the emotional, intellectual, and physical aspects of sexual attraction and expression. A person is born with his or her sexuality. Although it is a natural instinct, sexuality is greatly influenced by society. Every society considers some expressions of sexuality acceptable and others unacceptable. What is appropriate in the United States may not be appropriate in Egypt or China.

Several terms are related to sexuality, including **sex** and **gender**. Although people use them interchangeably, each has a specific meaning. The word *sex* describes a person's biological femaleness or maleness, including his or her genetic makeup and physical appearance. *Gender* describes one's femininity or masculinity based on psychological and social characteristics associated with being male or female. In the United States, for example, a male may feel he has to be strong and serve as the provider for his family. A female may feel she has to be nurturing and sensitive of others. Both sets of characteristics are psychological or social rather than biological.

GENDER IDENTITY

Most people develop a gender identity in the first few years of life, when they realize that they are male or female. Their gender identity, or personal sense of being male or female, includes their psychological perception of themselves as male or female. It is a self-label.

The formation of a gender identity is complicated. It begins at conception when one becomes genetically male or female. Each person receives one chromosome from the mother and one from the father. The mother always produces an X chromosome. If the father also produces an X, the baby is female. If he produces a Y, the baby is male. Therefore, the father always determines the sex of the baby.

Gender identity continues to form during early childhood, based on cultural influences. A **culture** is the way a group of people live, including their attitudes and values. It includes not only the things people make but also their ideas about themselves and others. Different cultures have different expectations for males and females. By about 18 months, a toddler has a good idea of what it means to be a boy or a girl.

Gender identity vs. biological sex

Sometimes one's biological sex does not match his or her gender identity. A person may have the physical anatomy of one sex but have feelings as if he or she belongs to the other sex.

People who are **transsexual** feel their biological sex does not match their gender identity. A transsexual may describe this feeling as being trapped in the wrong body. It is sometimes referred to as Gender Identity Disorder. Some transsexuals undergo **sex reassignment**—surgery to alter the appearance of their genitals to match the way they feel and hormone treatments to induce physical changes in the body. Those who seek the surgery are carefully screened for mental disorders and psychological health. After the surgery, they receive extensive counseling on how to live with their new identity. Despite these and other risks, the surgery allows some transsexuals to live in a physical body that matches their gender identity. Patients who make this decision come to realize that they are transsexual through experience. It doesn't happen overnight. Transsexuals may feel uneasy acting the way they are supposed to act and more comfortable acting like members of the other sex.

A similar term, **transgender,** describes the crossing of traditional gender lines because of discomfort with the gender roles generally accepted in one's society. Unlike transsexuals, a transgendered person does not feel trapped in the wrong body and has no desire to alter his or her genitals. A transgendered person's gender identity matches his or her biological sex, but he or she enjoys acting like the other sex at times. Some challenge the boundaries their culture places on one sex or the other by expressing their gender in forms considered by others to be inappropriate.

Some transgendered people engage in **cross-dressing.** Cross-dressing is wearing the clothing of a member of the other sex for sexual gratification. A man may wear women's clothing and feel better dressed as a woman.

GENDER ROLES

A **gender role** is the pattern of behavior a society considers acceptable for a particular sex. Family, peer groups, school, the media, and religion all influence preconceptions of gender roles. Together, they influence how people in a society think males and females should act.

Gender roles can be limiting. Expecting certain behaviors from one gender and other behaviors from another may limit the options an individual has. In the late 1800s and early 1900s, for example, women in the United States were barred from many occupations. They were also discouraged from holding jobs outside the home. During those years, men were discouraged from keeping the house or caring for children. Today those gender roles are changing. Many men and women are now freer to define their gender roles.

SEXUAL STEREOTYPING

Gender role expectations can lead to **stereotypes.** A stereotype is a label or judgment about an individual based on the characteristics of a group. These set opinions reduce individuals to categories and can lead to prejudice and discrimination.

In the United States, males are often stereotyped as tough and strong. Men and boys may feel they will be considered "sissies" if they cry or appear sensitive. Females are often stereotyped as nurturing and sensitive. Women may feel pressure to take care of the family rather than pursue careers. Many experts consider it important that both men and women express their emotions without being judged, choose the career of their choice, and live without restrictions based on their sex.

People today are becoming more **androgynous,** which means having characteristics of both sexes by presenting both masculine and feminine behaviors and traits in the same individual. Both men and women are realizing that they can break free from the stereotypes and live their lives the way they choose rather than what is socially expected. More couples in relationships are choosing what works for their individual, specific relationship.

Sexuality is influenced by a variety of factors. There is no right or wrong gender role or gender identity. It is important for people to feel comfortable about themselves and their relationships. Being an individual and breaking away from stereotypes can lead to happier, more fulfilling relationships both with oneself and with other people.

See also: Biology and Sex; Sexual Arousal

FURTHER READING

Colapinto, John. *As Nature Made Him: The Boy Who Was Raised a Girl.* New York: HarperCollins, 2006.

Lips, Hilary. *Sex and Gender: An Introduction.* Burr Ridge, Ill.: McGraw-Hill, 2004.

Strong, Bryan, Christine DeVault, Barbara W. Sayad, et al. *Human Sexuality: Diversity in Contemporary America.* New York: McGraw-Hill, 2004.

■ BIOLOGY AND SEX

The science of life and its divisions into gender—masculinity or femininity. Biology and sex include one's identification as male or female based on genetic makeup and anatomical sex characteristics. The body continually develops and changes as one ages. During the teen years, **puberty** occurs. Puberty is the stage of human development during which a child's body becomes sexually mature and develops into the adult form. By understanding their physical anatomy and changes associated with puberty, a teen is better able to understand his or her body and how it functions as a male or female.

PUBERTY

Adolescence is the stage of development between the start of puberty and the time an individual accepts full responsibility as an adult in society. During adolescence many physical and emotional changes take place. Although the average age for puberty is 12 for females and 14 for males, some individuals may experience changes as early as eight or nine.

For most teens, puberty is a tough time. Some don't know what to expect or when puberty will begin. Those who develop earlier than their friends may be embarrassed; those who are the last among their friends to develop may wonder if something is wrong with them.

In addition to the physical changes experienced by those who go through puberty early, the psychological effects can be troubling. Young girls who look older than they are may be pressured to act older. Unfortunately, when children are bombarded by sexual images and their bodies push them toward adulthood before they are psychologically ready, they lose the freedom to act like children.

The role of the gonads

When puberty occurs, a part of the brain called the **hypothalamus** increases certain secretions. The hypothalamus regulates body temperature, hunger, feelings of rage, aggression, pain, pleasure, and patterns of sexual arousal. The secretions from the hypothalamus cause the pituitary gland to release larger amounts of **hormones.** Hormones alter the activity of targeted cells of the body. These hormones stimulate the **gonads** to release more hormones. Gonads are the male and female sex glands, the testes and ovaries. **Testes** are the two male reproductive glands in which sperm and male sex hormones are produced. **Ovaries** are the two female reproductive organs in which egg cells develop and produce female sex hormones.

In males, testes produce **testosterone,** a hormone needed to produce sperm and for the development of male reproductive organs and body growth. In females, the ovaries release **estrogen,** a hormone needed to regulate the **menstrual cycle** and for the development of female reproductive organs and body growth. The menstrual cycle is the interaction of hormones that prepare a woman's body for possible pregnancy.

As males enter puberty, they may notice their testes becoming larger. Females in puberty may notice their breasts developing. As levels of hormones rise in both males and females, girls and boys begin to mature sexually.

Development of secondary sex characteristics

The visible changes that occur during puberty that distinguish males from females are known as **secondary sex characteristics.** The characteristics are considered secondary because they occur after the release of hormones.

In males, puberty causes hair growth on the face, under the arms, and in the pubic area. Pubic hair in males is usually the first sign of puberty. Males also begin to develop acne due to overactive oil glands, changes in their voices, development of muscles, and enlargement in their penises, scrotums, and testes. The **penis** consists of spongy tissue that becomes engorged with blood during sexual excitement, causing the organ to enlarge and become erect. The **scrotum** is the pouch of skin that contains the pair of testes.

Some of these changes may cause embarrassment. A male's voice may sometimes crack during puberty, a normal occurrence which indicates his voice is becoming deeper. Developing acne on the face can be another embarrassing change.

Q & A

Question: What's a "wet dream?"

Answer: The correct term for a wet dream is *nocturnal emission.* A wet dream occurs when a male ejaculates in his sleep. Some males wake up thinking they have wet the bed. Nocturnal emissions are a normal part of puberty. They indicate that a male can ejaculate and cause pregnancy.

In females, breast development is usually the first sign of puberty. Girls also develop hair on their legs, under their arms, and in the pubic area. Their hips get larger as do the **uterus, clitoris,** and **labia.** The uterus, an organ about the size of a fist, is the place where a fetus develops. The clitoris is the organ that is the center for sexual arousal in females. It is located above the **urethral opening** (the opening to the passageway through which urine passes from the body). The labia are folds of skin located on each side of the vagina. Females will also experience **menarche,** or their first menstrual period. Menarche usually occurs around age 12 or 13. Many girls do not have a regular period—one that occurs once a month—until several years after menarche.

The menstrual cycle
Menstruation is the monthly shedding of the uterine lining; blood and tissue leave the body through the vagina. Each month during

her menstrual cycle, a woman ovulates. Ovulation is the monthly release of an egg by an ovary. If the egg is not fertilized, menstruation occurs about 14 days later. Once a woman begins menstruating, she continues until she experiences menopause, or the ending of menstruation due to the aging process. The average age of menopause is 51. Since the ovaries produce estrogen and estrogen is needed for a menstrual cycle, menopause also occurs if the ovaries are surgically removed.

MALE SEXUAL ANATOMY AND PHYSIOLOGY

Anatomy is the structure of the body and the relationship of its parts to each other. The sexual anatomy of both males and females includes internal and external structures. Each has distinct functions. In males and females, the main purpose of one's sexual anatomy is reproduction (the process of producing a new individual).

External male sexual anatomy

The male external sexual anatomy includes the penis, scrotum, and testes. The penis is made up of nerves, blood vessels, and spongy and fibrous tissue. When a male becomes sexually aroused, the penis becomes erect, or hard, because it fills with blood. Sometimes a man cannot control his sexual arousal. Ejaculation is the process by which semen is forcefully expelled from the penis. Muscles at the base of the penis eject both semen and urine through the urethra, which runs lengthwise through the penis to the bladder. Semen and urine never pass through the urethra at the same time. The tip of the penis, known as the glans, is covered with a retractable piece of skin called the foreskin.

Q & A

Question: What is circumcision?

Answer: About 60 percent of male babies in the United States have their foreskin removed. This procedure is called a circumcision. According to the Centers for Disease Control and Prevention, several types of research have documented that male circumcision significantly reduces the risk of HIV. Many parents also have their sons circumcised so that their boys will look like other boys. However, when a man is erect, it is impossible to tell if he has been circumcised. Worldwide, about 30 percent of men are circumcised, of whom an estimated two-thirds are Muslim. Although families in most parts of the world do not circumcise their sons, most Americans do. Judaism is one of the few religions to require male circumcision, as well.

The **scrotum** helps to regulate the temperature of the testes for sperm production. The testes should be several degrees less than normal body temperature. To cool the testes when they are too warm, the scrotum stretches or hangs away from the body, and it tightens or pulls the testes closer to the body when they are too cold. It is normal for one testicle in the scrotal sac to hang lower than the other. At the back of each testicle is the **epididymis**. The epididymis is the comma-shaped organ that lies along the back of the testes. The epididymis is where sperm mature until they are ejaculated.

Q & A

Question: Why does my doctor check my testes for lumps?

Answer: Testicular cancer is most common in men ages 18–34. Many experts recommend that men check their testes regularly for lumps, which will feel similar to small, hard peas. Other signs of testicular cancer include:

- Any enlargement of a testicle
- A significant loss of size in one of the testicles
- A feeling of heaviness in the scrotum
- A dull ache in the lower abdomen or in the groin
- A sudden collection of fluid in the scrotum
- Pain or discomfort in a testicle or in the scrotum
- Enlargement or tenderness of the breasts

Internal male sexual anatomy

A male's internal sexual anatomy includes the **vas deferens, seminal vesicles, prostate gland,** and **Cowper's glands.** The vas deferens are long, thin tubes that carry sperm from each testicle to the urethra. The seminal vesicles are two small glands that produce most of the fluid in **semen** which provide nutrients to sperm.

Semen, also called seminal fluid, is the fluid that contains sperm discharged at ejaculation by a male through the penis. Semen contains about 200–500 million tiny sperm in each ejaculation. However, sperm only make up about 1 percent of the semen. The average amount of semen that comes out at each ejaculation is about one teaspoon.

The prostate gland produces some of the fluid in semen—about 30 percent—that nourishes and transports sperm. It is the size and shape of a walnut and is located at the base of the bladder. The Cowper's glands, located at each side of the urethra near the prostate gland, produce pre-ejaculatory fluid, also known as pre-cum, which may contain sperm.

FEMALE SEXUAL ANATOMY AND PHYSIOLOGY

Female sexual anatomy, like male sexual anatomy, includes both internal and external structures. Both of these structures aid in reproduction.

External female sexual anatomy

The external sexual anatomy, also known as the vulva, includes the **mons veneris, labia majora, labia minora,** clitoris, and urethral and vaginal openings. The mons veneris is the fatty tissue that protects the pubic bones. It becomes covered with hair during puberty. The labia majora are the outer lips of the vulva, and the labia minora are the inner lips.

The clitoris is located above the urethral opening where the labia minora meet. The urethral opening in females is below the clitoris and above the vaginal opening. The vaginal opening leads to the vagina. The area between the vaginal opening and the anus is called the **perineum.**

Fact Or Fiction?

Vaginal infections don't affect men.

The Facts: Females with a vaginal infection can pass it to a male through sexual intercourse. Although the male is not likely to have signs and symptoms, he, too, must be treated to prevent him from passing it back to his female partner once she is treated.

Internal female sexual anatomy

The internal structures of the female sexual anatomy include the vagina, cervix, uterus, fallopian tubes, and ovaries. The **vagina** serves as the birth canal. It is about three to five inches long, but expands and provides lubrication during arousal. The **cervix** is the opening to the uterus at the top of the vagina. Blood passes through the cervix during the menstrual cycle. This small opening is so tiny that only sperm can enter. (A woman can never lose a tampon or any other object inside of her body.)

The uterus is the organ that houses a fertilized egg which develops into a baby. The **fallopian tubes** are two tubes that extend from each side of the uterus to the ovaries. In the fallopian tubes, the egg and sperm meet and then travel to the uterus to implant.

If the fertilized egg implants in one of the fallopian tubes, an **ectopic pregnancy** may occur. An ectopic pregnancy is a pregnancy that occurs outside of the uterus, most commonly in the fallopian tube. This could rupture and cause uncontrolled bleeding, which is a serious medical emergency. Signs of an ectopic pregnancy include abdominal pain and spotting.

Finally, the ovaries are located at the end of each fallopian tube. The ovaries contain several hundred thousand immature ova, or eggs. Unlike men who produce sperm throughout their lives, women are usually born with all of their eggs.

Fact Or Fiction?

Women should have a Pap smear yearly beginning at age 21 or as soon as they become sexually active.

The Facts: The Pap smear is a test for cervical cancer administered yearly after age 21 or as soon as a woman becomes sexually active. The doctor lightly swabs the cervix with a long cotton swab collecting fluid from the cervix. This fluid is then sent to a lab for testing. During the visit, the doctor may also check the breasts for lumps, which could be indicative of breast cancer. This is also a time when many women discuss contraception with their doctor. Those who have had unprotected sex should ask for STD testing. (STD testing is not a regular part of a yearly pelvic exam.)

Although the male and female anatomy may seem different, they are similar in several ways. For each male organ, there is a similar female organ in tissue or function. For example, the vas deferens in the male are similar to the fallopian tubes in the female. The glans of the penis is much like the clitoris, and the testes can be compared to the ovaries.

Both males and females go through rapid periods of change during puberty, and both males and females play a part in reproduction. Knowing one's body will help to prepare a person to care for it and understand the way it functions.

See also: Conception, Pregnancy, and Childbirth

FURTHER READING

Bancroft, John, ed. *Sexual Development in Childhood.* Bloomington: Indiana University Press, 2003.

Steinberg, Laurence. *Adolescence.* 6th ed. Boston: McGraw-Hill, 2002.

■ BIRTH DEFECTS AND RISK-TAKING BEHAVIORS

Abnormalities that occur during fetal development and are present at birth. Although some birth defects are the result of genetic predisposition, others can be avoided by a woman's behavior while pregnant. Avoiding some risk-taking activity will help support both a healthy pregnancy and the birth of a healthy baby. Most birth defects occur during the first three months of pregnancy; the cause of up to 70 percent of birth defects is still unknown.

BIRTH DEFECTS

A birth defect may affect how the body looks, works, or both. It can be found before birth, at birth, or anytime after birth. Most defects are found within the first year of life. Some birth defects (such as cleft lip or clubfoot) are easy to see, but others (such as heart defects or hearing loss) are found using special tests (such as X rays, CAT scans, or hearing tests).

In the United States, about 3 percent of babies are born with birth defects, one every three minutes. Some defects can cause the baby to die, while others leave lasting effects on the baby's life. Babies with birth defects may need surgery or other medical treatments, but if they receive the help they need, these babies often lead full lives.

Fact Or Fiction?

Birth defects are the leading cause of infant mortality.

The Facts: Birth defects are the leading cause of infant deaths, accounting for more than 20 percent of all infant deaths, according to the Centers for Disease Control and Prevention (CDC). Birth defects affect about one in every 33 babies born in the United States each year. Seven to 10 percent of all children will require extensive medical procedures to diagnose or treat a birth defect. Babies born with a birth defect who survive have a greater chance of suffering from chronic illness and long-term disabilities than babies who are born healthy.

There are a number of things an expectant mother should avoid to help prevent birth defects. If taken when a woman is pregnant, certain drugs increase the chance of birth defects. Also, women who smoke and use alcohol while pregnant have a higher risk of having a baby with certain birth defects.

An expectant woman generally will do everything she can to ensure that she and her baby are well cared for during pregnancy. However, a genetic mutation, or an abnormal change in a **gene**, can cause a birth defect. There is no way for the mother to prevent such a mutation.

Some women have a higher chance of having a child with a birth defect. Women over the age of 35 have a higher chance of having a child with Down syndrome than women who are younger. A common genetic birth defect, Down syndrome is caused by the presence of all or part of an extra 21st **chromosome**. Researchers are unsure why age plays a factor in this mutation. Other women have a higher chance of having a baby with a birth defect because someone in their family had a similar problem. Other factors including obesity also affect the chances of having a baby with a birth defect.

Many doctors will recommend and provide genetic counseling, which usually includes screening of the parents to see if they are carriers of certain disorders. Genes tell each cell in the body how to combine with other cells to form parts of the body. For example, genes tell certain cells to make the heart, the kidneys, or the brain, and they tell other cells to make our physical features, like green eyes or brown hair. Genes also tell the cells how to work in the body. Genes give instructions for cells in our heart to beat, our stomach to digest food, our muscles to push and pull, and our brain to think. By having a screening, the family can find out the probability of their baby being born with a birth defect. Changes in single genes, groups of genes, or entire chromosomes can sometimes cause birth defects. These genetic changes might occur only in the infant, or they might have been passed down from one or both parents. Sometimes, there are other relatives in the family with the same birth defect, but not always. By knowing family history, genetic problems, heredity, and chronic diseases that family members have experienced, doctors are better able to provide useful information and appropriate medical care for expectant mothers.

Common birth defects, such as structural deformities of the heart, spina bifida, and Down syndrome, affect organs such as the heart, the nervous system, and the lips and mouth. Heart defects affect about one in every 100 to 200 babies, and some of these heart defects can be serious. A few are very severe, causing life-long conditions.

The common birth defect known as spina bifida affects the development of the spine and is seen in about one out of 1,000 pregnancies, making this neural defect fairly common. In the last several years, studies have proven that folic acid is a key component to preventing birth defects, particularly neural tube defects like spina bifida.

Birth defects known as orofacial clefts, including cleft lip, cleft palate, and combined cleft lip and cleft palate, are common defects of the lip and mouth. Cleft lip is more common than cleft palate. In many places around the world, orofacial clefts affect about one in 700 to 1,000 babies. Often these birth defects can be treated with reconstructive surgeries.

Q & A

Question: Does folic acid support the health of women of child-bearing age?

Answer: Yes, it is highly recommended by experts that women of childbearing age get at least 400 micrograms of folic acid every day.

Folic acid, also known as vitamin B9 or folate, is a nutrient known to prevent neural tube birth defects such as spina bifida. A daily dose of folic acid can be taken in the form of a multivitamin or through various food sources, including strawberries and oranges. The FDA is required to add folic acid to sources of grains as well, such as breakfast cereals and pastas. It's important to begin taking the folic acid before you are pregnant because most birth defects happen in the early stages of pregnancy.

RISKY BEHAVIORS TO AVOID

It is in the best interest of the expectant mother, as well as the baby, to seek the care of a medical professional before and during pregnancy. By making positive lifestyle choices including maintaining a healthy weight, eating well-balanced nutritional meals, and avoiding certain risky behaviors while pregnant, a baby's chances of being born with a birth defect are lowered. Drinking alcohol, smoking, and using illegal drugs should be avoided while pregnant. Also, a factor known as a *teratogen*, an environmental catalyst for birth defects, can include exposure to hazardous chemicals, rodents, cat feces, and certain prescription medications before and during pregnancy.

Alcohol

When a pregnant woman drinks alcohol, so does her baby. There is no known safe amount of alcohol to drink. According to the National Institute on Alcohol Abuse and Alcoholism, alcohol abuse during pregnancy is the leading preventable cause of mental retardation in offspring in the United States. When a pregnant woman drinks, she puts her baby at risk to develop fetal alcohol spectrum disorders, an umbrella term that classifies the level of mental, physical, and behavior problems as a result of drinking alcohol during pregnancy. The most severe of these disorders is fetal alcohol syndrome. Fetal alcohol syndrome affects the baby's physical and mental ability, resulting in abnormal facial features, growth deficiencies, and nervous system problems. The baby will also have problems with learning, memory, attention span, communication, vision, hearing, or a combination of these. Fetal Alcohol Syndrome is a permanent condition, so it is safest to avoid any alcohol during pregnancy.

Cigarettes

Smoking while pregnant causes prematurity, low birth rate, and susceptibility to sudden infant death syndrome (SIDS). Babies born of mothers who smoked while pregnant have a 30 percent chance of being born prematurely. The CDC reports that women who smoke during pregnancy are about twice as likely to experience problems with the development of the baby's membrane tissue and placenta. Smoking restricts the blood vessels, which restricts the amount of oxygen and nutrients the baby receives while in the womb.

Drugs

Illegal drugs such as cocaine are extremely harmful to the baby when a woman is pregnant. Just as smoking and alcohol directly affect development by inhibiting proper nutrients and oxygen from reaching the baby, so do street drugs. According to the American College of Obstetricians and Gynecology (ACOG), cocaine use during pregnancy increases the chance of premature labor by 25 percent. Babies can become addicted to the cocaine as well and will go through withdrawal symptoms once they are born. Some experts believe that learning difficulties may result as the child gets older. Defects of the genitals, kidneys, and brain are also possible.

Prescription Drugs

Always check with your health-care provider regarding prescribed medications that are being taken. A known medication that treats acne, Accutane (isotretinoin), should not be taken while pregnant due to the incidences of babies being born with defects. Other medications that are used to treat high blood pressure can also increase the chance of a baby being born with a birth defect.

Over-the-Counter Medicines

These are medicines that can be obtained without a prescription. The labels on **over-the-counter medications** provide helpful information for women who are pregnant and or nursing. Pain relievers such as ibuprofen or aspirin can cause problems with blood flow by increasing the chance for excessive bleeding during birth. As you would with prescription drugs, it is best to check with your health-care provider regarding taking over-the-counter medications.

Vaccines

The MMR vaccine is for measles, mumps, and rubella. If a woman gets one of these viruses while pregnant, it may cause her to have a miscarriage or to have a baby with birth defects. The MMR, like some other vaccines, is made with viruses that are alive but very weak. Because these viruses are alive, there is a very slight chance that they may cause harm to the baby. For this reason, a woman who may be pregnant should not get an MMR or other vaccine unless she is at high risk of getting a serious illness without it. She should talk about the risks and benefits of getting the vaccine with her doctor. A woman who learns she is pregnant soon after getting the vaccine should also talk with her doctor. Vaccines such as those for tetanus and hepatitis are made from dead viruses or parts of dead viruses and do not cause infection in the mother. These vaccines should not harm the fetus.

TEENS SPEAK

I'm the Visible Teen with the Invisible Disability

Nobody can see my disability. I look just like every other teenager—attractive, friendly, and talkative. But nobody sees my disability. They can't see how my neurons are scrambled in my brain. They can't see the misconnections between the left and right brain. They can't see the little empty spaces in my frontal lobes where brain cells were supposed to grow but didn't. Nobody knows that I have static encephalopathy because my mother drank when she was pregnant. But everybody can see how inappropriate my behavior can be when I am out in public. Everybody can see how immature I can be compared to other teenagers my age. When things have been too overwhelming for me, no one sees the two-year old tantrum as soon as I get home. I just want to be accepted and understood.

See also: Drugs, Alcohol, and Sex; Prenatal Care

FURTHER READING
Birth Defects Research for Children, Inc. Available online. URL: http://www.birthdefects.org. Accessed January 12, 2009.
Centers for Disease Control and Prevention. Available online. URL: http://www.cdc.gov/ncbddd/bd/default.htm. Accessed January 12, 2009.
Iannucci, Lisa. *Birth Defects, Diseases and People.* Berkeley Heights, N.J.: Enslow Publishers, 2000.

■ COMMUNITY, SUPPORT FROM THE

A group of people living in the same place under the same laws. Communities are bound together by common interests and standards. Members of a community recognize that what happens to one person in a community can affect everyone. Therefore many towns, cities, and even neighborhoods offer a variety of health services. These services include pregnancy testing, prenatal care, testing and treatment of sexually transmitted diseases (STDs), contraceptive aids, and general health exams.

HEALTH DEPARTMENTS

Health departments at both the city and county levels provide a variety of health-related services. Many provide STD testing, prenatal care, and health exams as well as treatment. If a health department is unable to help with a particular problem, they will usually provide a referral.

PLANNED PARENTHOOD

Planned Parenthood is a reproductive health care organization that has chapters throughout the nation. Founded in 1916 as a nonprofit organization, Planned Parenthood offers a variety of services, including sexual health education and information on teen sexual health issues such as dating and relationships, sexually transmitted diseases, pregnancy, prenatal care, and contraceptive use.

Many Planned Parenthood chapters provide pamphlets on these issues stressing the importance of preventing STDs and unplanned pregnancy. In addition, many local chapters of Planned Parenthood have created health-related programs or services for their community based on the specific needs of that community.

Although Planned Parenthood is often thought of as an abortion clinic, abortions are only a small part of the services that the organization offers. Planned Parenthood also provides pelvic exams, contraception, emergency contraception, and STD testing and treatment. These centers offer a variety of services related to sexual health for both men and women.

Q & A

Question: How much does it cost to get tested for an STD?

Answer: Most clinics charge a small fee for STD testing. Some set their fees on a sliding scale, based on one's salary or income. Therefore, someone who does not have a job or has a small income pays less than someone who makes more money. There are some clinics that conduct free STD testing. Check with your local health department to learn where free STD testing is provided in your community. Health departments of a community are usually listed in the local phone book.

RAPE CRISIS CENTERS

Most communities have a rape crisis center that offers emotional support and comfort to survivors of **rape,** the crime of forcing a person to have sexual intercourse against his or her will. According to RAINN: The Rape Abuse & Incest National Network, one in six women and one in 33 men will be sexually assaulted in their lifetime. People working at rape crisis centers are trained to help victims after an attack.

Many rape crisis centers send a crisis worker to sit with the survivor of the rape during her exam at the hospital. The worker can explain what to expect during the exam and can help the survivor feel more comfortable. If the survivor decides to report the rape to police, the rape crisis worker will provide assistance in locating legal services. Just because a woman goes to a rape crisis center does not mean she has to report the rape to the police.

Some rape crisis centers also provide educational programs to make the entire community more aware of the dangers of sexual assaults, to advise ways to prevent such assaults, and to inform people on how to report rape and the importance of doing so.

WOMEN'S SHELTERS

Many communities have shelters for abused or neglected women and their children. According to the Centers for Disease Control and Prevention (CDC), in 2006, one in 11 adolescents reported being a victim of physical dating violence. Each year, 4.8 million women are raped or physically assaulted by an intimate partner—a husband, dating partner, or live-in boyfriend. Of all women, 17.6 percent are victims of rape. Of the women raped, 44 percent, are under age 18.

With these high rates of sexual and physical abuse toward women, shelters can be critical in saving a life by protecting a woman from physical harm. They also provide food, clothing, and other necessities.

Q & A

Question: How can I find a women's shelter in my community for my mom and me?

Answer: You won't find listings for women's shelters in the phone book. Often, these shelters are group homes located inconspicuously in neighborhoods. The homes must be anonymous to protect the women they're housing from abusive partners. To find help in your area, call the National Domestic Violence Hotline at (800) 656-HOPE.

ADOPTION SERVICES

A number of communities provide adoption services for pregnant females who may not want to be mothers or those who are unable to support a child. Instead of ending the pregnancy, they continue the pregnancy and then turn the baby over to another person or family to raise.

Those wishing to adopt a child have two options. They can contact a state-licensed adoption agency, an organization that seeks safe and stable homes for babies put up for adoption, or they can seek an independent or private adoption with the help of an attorney or physician. Although the process can be quite lengthy, often lasting several years for the adoptive parents, a state-licensed agency may be the best option for someone who wishes to adopt an older child or a child with special needs.

Those who wish to adopt a baby often make their own arrangements with a woman willing to give up custody of her child. An attorney is often necessary to protect the rights of all parties involved. Each state has its own laws concerning independent adoptions. Prospective parents need to know their own state laws as well as the state laws of the birth mother.

HIV/AIDS CLINICS

According to the CDC, AIDS is the second leading cause of death among people between the ages of 25 and 44. Only injuries kill more people in this age range. AIDS stands for acquired immunodeficiency syndrome, a chronic disease caused by HIV, the human immunodeficiency virus in which the immune system is weakened and unable to fight infections.

The CDC estimates that more than a million people in the United States and 40 million people worldwide are infected with either HIV or AIDS. Many communities provide testing, support, and treatment for those who are HIV positive. Some communities have clinics devoted solely to those with HIV/AIDS. Others may offer the same services through other agencies such as the health department or a physician's office.

Some clinics offer **anonymous testing** and **confidential testing**. With anonymous testing, each person is given a number. The individual's name never appears with the results. Confidential testing means that one's name is listed with the results. However, those results will not be made public. Some consider confidential testing to be less private than anonymous testing. The CDC keeps track of all positive HIV tests conducted through confidential testing.

WOMEN'S CENTERS IN HOSPITALS

Almost every hospital has a women's center. These centers provide a variety of sexual-health services. These typically include STD testing, pelvic exams, counseling, prenatal care, parenting education, general health education, rape and sexual assault support, and more.

COUNSELING

Counseling services are also available to many individuals. Counselors are trained to work with individuals and groups to help them discover their own needs and work through problems. Although counseling services can be expensive, many insurance plans will help to pay for them. People seek counselors to address stress and anxiety in their lives, work through a difficult event such as a rape, learn to manage their weight, or break an unhealthy addiction such as drinking.

FINDING THE RIGHT SUPPORT

Many services are available in the community to assist people dealing with a variety of sexual health issues. When seeking community assistance, one should find a provider who is professional, courteous, and compassionate. Most sexual health providers believe strongly in what they do and try to make their clients feel comfortable. Providers should not judge people, but rather do their best to support those in need. If a person has a negative experience with one provider, he or she should look for another provider who makes him or her comfortable. Most people in these areas are passionate about helping others deal with sexual-health issues.

See also: Dating; Sex and the Law

FURTHER READING

Centers for Disease Control and Prevention. "HIV/AIDS in the U.S." Available online. URL: http://www.cdc.gov/HIV/resources. Accessed January 12, 2009.

■ CONCEPTION, PREGNANCY, AND CHILDBIRTH

Conception, the fusion of the egg and sperm. The process results in a fertilized egg which develops into a **fetus**. A fetus is the stage of life from two months after conception to birth. The (approximately) 40 weeks during which the fetus develops is called pregnancy, and it ends with childbirth the process of giving birth to a baby.

During pregnancy, a woman may think about childbirth. Although there is some risk involved, childbirth usually results in a healthy baby and mother. Most women experience pregnancy as a relatively comfortable and joyous time. By taking care of her body and receiving regular checkups with her doctor during pregnancy, a woman can help minimize the risk of possible complications.

FERTILIZATION

Each month a woman's body releases an egg from an **ovary**, the female reproductive organ. This process is called **ovulation**. Once the egg is released, it travels through a **fallopian tube,** one of two tubes that extend from each side of the **uterus** to the ovaries. The uterus is a hollow muscular organ in which the fertilized egg develops. Once an egg is released from an ovary, it is viable—alive and able to be fertilized—for approximately 12–48 hours. If an egg is not fertilized, it is expelled along with the uterine lining during **menstruation.** Menstruation is the monthly loss of blood and tissue lining the uterus if no fertilized egg is present.

Sperm, the male reproductive cells, are released into a woman's vagina during intercourse. The **vagina,** which encompasses the penis during sexual intercourse, is the passage leading from the external female genitals to the internal reproductive organs. It is also the pathway or birth canal through which the baby is born. Sperm are viable in a woman's body for approximately 48 hours, although some may be viable for up to five days. For fertilization to occur, intercourse should take place within five days before and one day after ovulation.

Once sperm enter a woman's vagina, they swim past the **cervix,** the end of the uterus opening toward the vagina, through the uterus, and into the fallopian tubes. Although many sperm may reach the egg, only one is able to enter. When a sperm enters the egg, the two form a **zygote,** a single cell from which a child develops.

In the course of the next few days, the zygote travels through the fallopian tube to the uterus. At about day four or five after fertilization, the zygote enters the uterus. There the zygote implants itself in the lining of the uterus and is now called the **blastocyst.** This stage of development lasts between the time the fertilized egg has implanted itself in the uterus—about day six to day 14. The blastocyst rapidly grows into an **embryo,** which then develops in the uterus from week two through week eight. At week eight, the embryo is called a **fetus.**

Fact Or Fiction?

There are only certain times of the month when a woman can get pregnant.

The Facts: A woman usually ovulates—or releases an egg—once a month, around day 14 of her menstrual cycle. Day 14 is about two weeks after the first day of the woman's period. At this time, an egg is most likely to be in the fallopian tube to meet a possible sperm. Sperm can usually live in a woman's body for approximately 72 hours (3 days). Therefore, a woman is most likely to get pregnant a few days before and after ovulation.

Signs of pregnancy

Some signs of pregnancy include missing a period, breast tenderness, fatigue, frequent urination, and **morning sickness** (feelings of nausea and vomiting early in pregnancy). Morning sickness can occur at any time of the day or night; however, it is most likely to occur when the pregnant woman does not have food in her stomach. Not every pregnant woman experiences morning sickness, but eating healthy snacks throughout the day can relieve some of the symptoms for those who do.

If a woman believes she is pregnant, she may decide to take a home pregnancy test. Home tests check a woman's urine for the hormone **human chorionic gonadotropin** (HCG). HCG is released when the fertilized egg implants in the uterus. Since implantation takes about a week, the test is not effective until at least seven days after intercourse. Home pregnancy tests are available at most drugstores and supermarkets.

Q & A

Question: Where do twins come from?

Answer: Fertilization occurs when a single sperm enters one egg and develops into a baby. If the fertilized egg splits into two, **identical twins** are formed. They are identical because they come from the same egg and sperm, so they have the same **genes**, or biological units of heredity. If a female releases two eggs, both may be fertilized with a separate sperm. These twins are called **fraternal twins** and do not look identical.

FETAL DEVELOPMENT

Although many people think a pregnancy lasts nine months, a pregnancy usually lasts about 40 weeks, closer to 10 months. The pregnancy is divided into three trimesters, each about three months long.

The first trimester

The first trimester begins with fertilization of the egg. Growth is rapid during the first three months. The arms, legs, eyes, fingers, and toes all begin to form. The fetus, which already has fingerprints, can squint, swallow, and wrinkle its forehead. During the third month, the heart begins to beat. Other internal organs also begin to function. The fetus is now three inches long. It sleeps and wakes. It also exercises its muscles by turning its head, curling its toes, and opening and closing its mouth.

The second trimester

The second trimester begins in the fourth month of pregnancy. By now, the mother feels movements and the fetus's weight has increased to one pound. By month six, the fetus is about 10–12 inches long, with clearly formed fingernails, eyebrows, eyelashes, and possibly hair. By the end of this trimester, the fetus can hear and has opened its eyes.

The third trimester

During the third trimester the fetus increases in weight from about four pounds in month seven to over seven pounds at birth. It grows from about 12 inches during month seven to about 20 inches in month nine. The skin is covered in **vernix,** a waxy, protective substance.

PRENATAL CARE

Prenatal care, the care a woman receives during pregnancy, is designed to ensure the health of the baby. Prenatal care includes proper nutrition, regular checkups, and exercise. It also means avoiding smoking or drinking alcohol. Whatever goes into a pregnant woman's body can possibly affect her baby. Since pregnancy can be a very emotional experience, taking time to relax quietly when pregnant may also be beneficial.

Nutrients are required for the formation of new cells and the development of organs in the fetus. All of the baby's nutrients come from the mother. Therefore a pregnant woman may need to eat more food and healthier food. If a pregnant woman eats nutritious meals during her pregnancy, she is more likely to have a healthy baby.

Regular checkups are essential to help ensure the health of the developing fetus and the expectant mother. According to the Centers for Disease Control and Prevention (CDC), the more prenatal care a woman receives, the fewer problems she has with her pregnancy and delivery. In addition, the infant is more likely to be born healthy. Regular check-

DID YOU KNOW?

Women's Nutritional Needs: Recommended Daily Allowances for Females, Ages 25–50

	Nonpregnant	Pregnant	Breast-feeding
Protein (grams)	50	60	65
Vitamin A (µg [micrograms])	800	800	1,300
Vitamin D (µg)	5	10	10
Vitamin E (mg [milligrams])	8	10	12
Vitamin C (mg)	60	70	95
Thiamine (mg)	1.1	1.5	1.6
Riboflavin (mg)	1.3	1.6	1.8
Niacin (mg)	15	17	20
Vitamin B 6 (mg)	1.6	2.2	2.1
Folacin (folate) (mg)	180	400	280
Vitamin B 12 (µg)	2	2.2	2.6
Calcium (mg)	800	1,200	1,200
Phosphorus (mg)	800	1,200	1,200
Magnesium (mg)	280	320	355
Iron (mg)	15	30	15
Zinc (mg)	12	19	19
Iodine (µg)	150	175	200

Source: National Academy of Sciences National Research Council, 2006.

ups can alert the doctor to possible illnesses during pregnancy such as high blood pressure, **toxemia**, and **diabetes**. Toxemia, or pre-eclampsia or eclampsia, depending on severity, is an abnormally high blood pressure and fluid retention. Diabetes is a disease in which the body does not produce or properly use insulin, the hormone needed to convert sugar and other foods into energy.

During pregnancy, regular exercise increases energy levels, promotes emotional well-being, and boosts the immune system. Physical activity also helps prepare a pregnant woman for childbirth, which is physically demanding. She may also return to her pre-pregnancy shape more quickly after delivery if she continues to exercise throughout her pregnancy.

The CDC recommends that pregnant women give up smoking, because smoking slows the fetus's growth. Women who smoke are also more likely to have a miscarriage, a baby with a cleft lip and palate, or a **low-birth-weight** (LBW) baby (a baby weighing less than 5.5 pounds at birth). Babies of mothers who smoke are also at a greater risk of **sudden infant death syndrome** (SIDS), the mysterious death of an apparently healthy infant during sleep. Exposing a baby to secondhand smoke can also increase his or her risk of SIDS.

Q & A

Can my girlfriend smoke while she's pregnant if she cuts back to a few cigarettes a day?

Answer: Smoking while a woman is pregnant can lead to a low-birth-weight baby and other serious health problems. Smoking also increases a woman's chance of a miscarriage. Since smoking reduces the amount of oxygen in the blood, the baby's growth can be slowed down. Babies born to mothers who smoke are also at increased risk of a cleft lip and palate. Secondhand smoke is also dangerous. Infants who are around smokers are more likely to have respiratory problems throughout their lives.

Drinking alcohol while pregnant is also dangerous to the baby. The baby experiences the same amount of alcohol that the mother does. However, it stays in the baby's system longer than it stays in the mother's. Women who drink during pregnancy are also putting their babies at an increased risk of **fetal alcohol syndrome** (FAS), a serious condition that can cause mental retardation and facial malformation as well as growth and development problems. The CDC estimates that about one to two in every 1,000 infants born in the United States has FAS.

Drugs should be avoided during pregnancy. A pregnant woman should clear even over-the-counter drugs like cold medicines with a doctor before taking them. Even tiny amounts of nicotine, tobacco, alcohol, and drugs can cause damage to the fetus.

TEENS SPEAK

I Drank During My Pregnancy

I didn't know I was pregnant until the end of my first trimester. I didn't have a period, but I didn't think anything of it because my periods are irregular. I know alcohol is bad for a baby, but I had no idea I was pregnant. When I was at my boyfriend's party last month, I got drunk and threw up. Once I found out I was pregnant, I panicked. I won't touch alcohol again while I'm pregnant.

I know about fetal alcohol syndrome and was so scared I had hurt my baby. I talked to my doctor about it, and we decided to run some tests. We also talked about the chances of miscarriage and other possible problems that result from drinking while pregnant. I was pretty nervous while getting the tests. Luckily my tests came back OK.

I was lucky. As far as we can tell my baby is healthy. I won't drink again now that I know I'm pregnant. It's not worth the risk. I'd hate to think that I caused my own baby to be mentally or physically disabled. It's not worth it!

CHILDBIRTH

A few weeks before childbirth, **lightening** occurs. During lightening, the baby lowers itself in the uterus in preparation for birth, making room for the mother to breathe more easily. At this time, most babies are positioned head-down. A mother may also feel uterine contractions called **Braxton-Hicks** contractions, which occur in preparation for labor.

Labor occurs in three stages. The first stage begins with contractions, the tightening of the uterine muscles to push the baby out, and ends when the cervix is fully dilated at 10 centimeters. The cervix dilates, or expands, to allow the baby to pass through. The first stage is the longest, usually lasting 10 to 16 hours for a woman's first childbirth. Some women experience their **water breaking,** and others won't. When a woman's water breaks, the **amniotic sac** ruptures in preparation for birth. The amniotic sac is a thin protective membrane surrounded with fluid to protect the developing fetus. Many women feel their water breaking as well as the **mucus plug** leaving their body. The mucus plug is the tissue and blood that cover the cervix during pregnancy to protect the fetus.

The second stage of labor begins when the cervix is fully dilated and ends with the delivery of the baby. This stage can last from 30 minutes to two or more hours. During this time, a woman can actively push with each contraction. Pain can be intense during the pushing phase, so discussing options for pain relief with a doctor prior to delivery is important. Once the baby is born, a physician quickly checks his or her color and breathing. The **umbilical cord,** which connects the fetus to the placenta, is clamped off several inches from the baby's belly button. The infant begins to breathe on its own immediately after delivery.

The third stage of labor involves the birth of the placenta. It is usually expelled within 30 minutes of delivery of the baby and, with one or two contractions, comes out easily.

Cesarean section
According to the National Center for Health Statistics, about 30.3 percent of all babies are delivered by **cesarean section,** the removal of the baby through an incision in the abdominal wall and uterus. A physician may recommend a cesarean section for reasons related to the baby, such as abnormalities in the development of the fetus or an abnormal fetal heart rate pattern. It may also be called for if there are signs that the baby is in an abnormal position within the uterus or there are multiple babies.

Some cesarean sections are required for reasons related to the mother, including heart disease, pre-eclampsia, or eclampsia. A cesarean section is also likely to be called for if the mother has a genital herpes infection, an HIV infection, or had previous surgery in the uterus.

Problems with labor or delivery may also result in a cesarean section. Those problems may include a long labor, a baby with a head too large to pass through the mother's pelvis, and problems with the placenta or umbilical cord.

The postpartum period
Childbirth and infant care can be physically and emotionally exhausting. Many women experience temporary sadness and emotional upset after having a baby due to sudden emotional, physical, and hormonal changes. These changes also cause many women to experience tired-

ness, loneliness, or fear. This period is often called the **baby blues** and usually goes away within a few days of having a baby.

Although less common, some women experience **postpartum depression** after having a baby. Postpartum depression is a form of depression thought to be related to hormonal changes following the delivery of a child. This depression may include insomnia, anxiety, panic attacks, and hopelessness. In severe cases, thoughts of death or suicide may occur. During the postpartum period, the body is slowly starting to return to normal, and hormone levels drop rapidly. It is important for a new mother experiencing this to see a doctor if the depression continues, or if she has thoughts about hurting herself or her baby.

Bleeding and discharge to rid the body of no-longer-needed uterine tissue usually occurs several weeks after delivery. A woman should wait four to six weeks after having a baby to have intercourse again. These weeks are needed for the body to heal.

Q & A

Question: What are the benefits of breast-feeding?

Answer: Breast-feeding, or nursing, provides the best nutrients for a baby. Breast-feeding provides a baby with antibodies to protect against infection. It also helps the mother and baby bond.

During the first few days following delivery, the mother produces **colostrum,** a clear substance rich in antibodies. Milk is produced a few days later.

Doctors recommend breast-feeding for up to six months to a year. However, some mothers are not able to breast-feed. Although most people believe breast-feeding comes naturally and is easy to do, it can be difficult to learn, and even painful during the first few weeks. Nurses can provide tips on making it easier. Mothers who breast-feed should drink plenty of water and eat a healthy diet. In addition, a mother needs extra calories when breast-feeding. Breast-feeding also helps the mother lose weight and return to her previous size more quickly and is an economical way to nourish a baby.

Pregnancy and childbirth can be great experiences, especially if the pregnant woman takes care of her body and seeks prenatal care.

By knowing the signs of pregnancy and childbirth, a woman will feel more prepared and at ease.

See also: Biology and Sex; Birth Defects and Risk-Taking Behaviors; Prenatal Care

FURTHER READING

Eisenberg, Arlene, Heidi Murkoff, and Sandee Hathaway. *What to Expect When You're Expecting.* 4th ed. New York: Workman Publishing, 2008.

Elise-Weiss, Robin. *The Everything Pregnancy Fitness Book.* Cincinnati: Adams Median, 2006.

Stoppard, Miriam. *Dr. Miriam Stoppard's New Pregnancy & Birth Book.* New York: Ballantine Books, 2000.

▄ CONTRACEPTIVES INVOLVING RISK

Although there are many contraceptives currently available that are effective, some couples rely on methods that do not significantly reduce the risk of pregnancy. An effective method is one proven to work when used correctly. A method involving risk is one that is not proven to prevent pregnancy—despite popular beliefs.

WITHDRAWAL

One risky method of contraception is **withdrawal,** or pulling out. A man withdraws his penis just before **ejaculation,** the process by which semen is forcefully expelled from the penis. This method requires that the male have great control over his body. Withdrawal is also risky because there may be sperm in the **pre-ejaculatory fluid,** or pre-cum, the fluid that may come out of the penis during sexual arousal before ejaculation. Not only sperm, but also sexually transmitted diseases (STDs) may be present in pre-ejaculatory fluid.

Even if sperm are not ejaculated into the vagina, pregnancy is possible if sperm are released near the vaginal opening. Sperm can travel along any fluid near the vaginal opening and enter the vagina. Withdrawal also can affect a couple's sexual pleasure since a man will be thinking about when to withdraw, and a woman will be concerned that he does it on time.

Q & A

Question: Can I get my girlfriend pregnant if I don't ejaculate inside her?

Answer: Yes. Even if a male ejaculates outside a woman's vagina, he may still have sperm in his **urethra** during intercourse. The urethra is the tube through which urine passes from the bladder to outside the body. In males, the urethra also acts as a passageway for sperm. Sperm may enter the vagina through the pre-ejaculatory fluid that is released to lubricate the vagina during intercourse. It is important to always use a contraceptive from the beginning to the end of intercourse.

TEENS SPEAK

My Girlfriend Asked Me to "Pull Out"

My girlfriend and I have been dating a little over a year. We're 17 and decided to have sex about a month ago. The first few times I wore a condom. I was comfortable with that, and I felt I was protecting her from getting pregnant. Even though I trust her, I still worry about STDs. With a condom, I felt protected.

One night she said she wanted to try it without a condom. Some of her friends told her it felt better without one. She told me I could just pull out. The idea made me totally nervous. Even though I love her and want to make her happy, I know it is risky. I wasn't sure I'd be able to control myself in the heat of the moment. She said if I loved her I should want to show her. I told her I loved her completely but still wanted to wear a condom. I reminded her that neither of us was ready to be a parent, and she agreed. Even though it might feel better without a condom, that is something we can look forward to if we really do stay together forever.

FERTILITY AWARENESS METHODS

Fertility awareness methods of contraception rely on knowing exactly when a woman is most fertile. Each of these methods tries to pinpoint **ovulation** (the moment a woman releases an egg) to avoid unprotected intercourse during the time she is most likely to conceive. Even though these methods have no side effects and cost nothing, their disadvantages greatly outweigh their advantages.

The main problem with this method is that knowing the exact time of ovulation can be difficult. Many females have irregular **menstrual cycles,** the hormonal interactions that prepare a woman's body for possible pregnancy. The timing of ovulation may also change due to illness or stress. Not surprisingly, the overall failure rate of these methods is about 20–25 percent, according to Planned Parenthood. Many couples also find these methods inconvenient. They do not keep accurate records of the woman's menstrual cycle or find the period of abstinence during her "unsafe" days too long. Some don't like the idea of having to plan when to have sex. Three of the most popular fertility awareness methods are based on the calendar, cervical mucus, and body temperature.

Rhythm or calendar method

The **rhythm method,** also known as the calendar method, involves counting days in a woman's menstrual cycle. To avoid pregnancy, a woman should not have intercourse several days before, during, and after ovulation. Generally she cannot have sex for a week, since it is impossible to determine exactly when ovulation begins and sperm can live in a woman's body for up to 72 hours, or three days.

To calculate the day of ovulation using the rhythm method, the first day of a female's period is considered day one. This day is the beginning of her menstrual cycle. Fourteen days later is the day she is most likely to ovulate if she has a regular cycle. However, many women don't have regular cycles, so it is almost impossible to know when a particular woman is ovulating. Many teens do not yet have a regular menstrual cycle, making the rhythm method an unreliable choice.

Cervical mucus method

Another fertility awareness method is based on changes in the female's **cervical mucus,** the naturally occurring mucus produced by the **cervix.** The cervix is a small opening to the **uterus,** the hollow organ in which the fetus develops. The mucus becomes thicker and stringy during ovulation, the time when a woman is most fertile. Taking note of these changes can help to identify when a woman is ovulating. She can check her mucus by wiping herself each time she uses the toilet to observe secretions on the tissue. She can also observe discharge in her underpants.

Changes in the color, amount, and consistency of mucus occur during a woman's menstrual cycle. After menstruation there are usually a few dry days. This time is considered a safe period in which to have intercourse without risk of pregnancy. Prior to ovulation, a yellow or white sticky discharge occurs. Avoiding unprotected intercourse during this time is important. Several days later, around day 14, clear, stringy, and stretchy mucus, similar to an egg white, appears. A woman feels lubrication or wetness, the vagina's way of preparing for sperm. About four or five days later—day 18 or 19—the mucus becomes cloudy and the risk of getting pregnant is reduced.

Relying on changes in cervical mucus is risky because douching, vaginal infections, semen, medications, lubrication from sexual arousal, and contraceptive foams and jellies can interfere with the natural flow of mucus. Some women track the mucus for at least a month before using it as a fertility awareness method. According to Planned Parenthood, the failure rate with this method is about 20 percent.

Body temperature method

A third fertility awareness method involves keeping records of a woman's body temperature to pinpoint ovulation. She takes her temperature each day usually before getting out of bed in the morning.

Body temperature usually drops slightly just before ovulation and rises one degree after ovulation due to changes in hormone levels. If the woman's temperature has slightly risen for three days in a row, she can assume she has ovulated. The body temperature method has a failure rate of at least 20 percent.

Q & A

Question: Can you get pregnant when you are nursing a baby?

Answer: Some people believe you can't get pregnant while nursing a baby, because women do not ovulate for some time after childbirth. If a woman breast-feeds her infant, the hormones involved in nursing may delay ovulation a little longer. However, a woman has no way of knowing when she will begin ovulating again. Ovulation occurs *before* a woman has her period. So, there is a chance she could ovulate and get pregnant again before actually having a period.

PREVENTING PREGNANCY

Although some people rely on risky contraceptive methods, using a proven method—one recommended by doctors—is a better choice. Using one of the natural methods along with another effective method may be beneficial. For instance, any time a woman can avoid intercourse around ovulation, her risk of becoming pregnant is reduced.

Experts suggest that couples always question the effectiveness of contraceptive methods. Unless a method is proven effective, some risk is involved.

See also: Conception, Pregnancy, and Childbirth; Contraceptives: Practices Proven Safe; Relationships and Responsibilities

FURTHER READING

Hatcher, Robert, Anita Nelson, and Miriam Zieman. *A Pocket Guide to Managing Contraception.* Tiger, Ga.: Bridging the Gap Communications, 2004.

Kass-Annesse, Barbara, and Hal Danzer. *The Fertility Awareness Workbook.* Atlanta: Printed Matter, 1990.

McLaren, Angus. *A History of Contraception.* Oxford: Basil Blackwell, 1991.

■ CONTRACEPTIVES: PRACTICES PROVEN SAFE

Methods of proven reliability used to prevent **conception,** the fusion of the egg and sperm that results in pregnancy. Although couples have a variety of effective contraceptives to choose from, they should keep in mind that no contraceptive method is 100 percent effective, other than abstinence. Contraceptives must be used correctly and consistently to be effective. The main types of contraceptives are hormonal methods, barrier methods, intrauterine devices (IUDs), and sterilization. Each has its benefits and its drawbacks.

HORMONAL METHODS

Some birth control methods work by altering **hormone** levels. Hormones are chemical substances that act as messengers within the body regulating various functions. Hormonal methods stop **ovulation,** the release of an egg that can be fertilized. They may also thicken the **cervical mucus,** the naturally occurring mucus secreted by the cervix,

DID YOU KNOW?

Effectiveness of Proven Contraception Methods

Method	Effectiveness if used correctly	Typical number out of 100 who become pregnant accidentally*
Combination birth control pill	99.7%	8
Contraceptive patch	99%	8
Vaginal contraceptive ring	99%	8
Depo-Provera	99.7%	3
Lunelle	99.5%	3
Male condoms	98%	15
Female condoms	95%	21
Diaphragm with spermicide	94%	16
Cervical cap	91%	16
IUD	99%	2

*Number of women out of 100 who become pregnant by the end of the first year of using a method.

Source: Strong, Bryan, Christine DeVault, Barbara W. Sayad, et al. *Human Sexuality: Diversity in Contemporary America*. New York. McGraw-Hill, 2004.

to prevent the entry of sperm. The **cervix** is the opening to the **uterus** (the hollow organ in which a fetus develops). In addition, hormonal methods may also thin the lining of the uterus to inhibit implantation of the fertilized egg.

Although hormonal contraceptives protect against unwanted pregnancy, they do not protect against sexually transmitted diseases (STDs). In addition, few are reliable during the first month of use. Women should always use a backup method during the first month they take a hormonal contraceptive.

Birth control pill

Since their approval in the 1960s, the birth control pill has been the most commonly used form of contraception in the United States. Over

30 different brands are available, all containing similar amounts of **estrogen** and **progesterone,** or just progesterone.

Estrogen is the principal female hormone that regulates the hormonal interactions that prepare a woman's body for pregnancy. Progesterone is also a female hormone. It affects many aspects of the female body, including the **menstrual cycle** (the hormonal interactions that prepare a woman's body for possible pregnancy).

Although pills containing both estrogen and progesterone are most commonly prescribed, the **minipill** contains only progesterone. This birth control pill is generally prescribed for women who should not take estrogen for health reasons or because they are nursing. Estrogen can dry up a nursing mother's milk. This minipill is slightly less effective than combination birth control pills and must be taken precisely as prescribed.

Fact Or Fiction?

If a woman forgets to take a birth control pill, she needs to use a backup method to prevent pregnancy.

The Facts: Birth control pills must be taken every day at about the same time. If a woman forgets to take a pill, she should take it as soon as she remembers and then take the next pill at the regular time. As a result, she may take two pills in one day but will not need to use a backup method. However, if she skips two days of pills she should use a backup method. She should first take two pills on the day she remembers and two pills the following day. From then on, she can continue to take one a day.

The advantages of the pill include an effectiveness rate of over 95 percent. It is relatively inexpensive and reversible. A woman can take the pill for any length of time without having difficulty getting pregnant in the future. The pill may also regulate a woman's menstrual cycle, reduce menstrual flow and menstrual cramps, enlarge breast size, and reduce acne. In addition, the pill reduces the risk of ovarian and endometrial cancers.

One disadvantage of the pill is the need for a prescription from a doctor. The pill must also be taken every day around the same time.

Possible side effects include nausea, vomiting, weight gain, and depression. The pill is not recommended for smokers, because a combination of smoking and estrogen may result in blood clots, which can cause heart attacks and strokes. Most important, the pill does not protect the woman from sexually transmitted diseases.

Emergency contraceptive pill

The emergency contraceptive pill is a high-dose birth control pill given twice within 72 hours of having unprotected sex. One pill is taken as soon as possible and the second pill 12 hours later. If a couple uses a defective condom or no contraception at all, the emergency contraceptive pill can prevent an unwanted pregnancy. It works by inhibiting or delaying ovulation, altering the transport of eggs and/or sperm, or inhibiting implantation of a fertilized egg.

There are two types of emergency contraception pill available: Preven contains both estrogen and progesterone; Plan B contains only progesterone. Nausea and vomiting, irregular bleeding, and breast tenderness are potential side effects. However, Plan B is less likely to cause nausea, because it does not contain estrogen.

Emergency contraception is not an abortion pill. It does not affect a fertilized egg already attached to the wall of the uterus. Therefore, an emergency contraception pill will not harm a developing fetus if taken by a woman who is already pregnant. However, emergency contraception should not be used as birth control. It is currently available without a prescription nationwide to individuals age 17 and above; it is available to those under 17 by prescription.

Contraceptive patch

Approved in 2001, the **contraceptive patch,** called Ortho Evra, is a one-inch square that can be worn anywhere on the body. Most women attach the patch to their hip, lower back, shoulder, or some other spot that cannot easily be seen. The patch prevents pregnancy by releasing a dose of estrogen and progesterone similar to the dose in a week's supply of birth control pills. A woman wears one patch a week for three weeks. She does not wear one during her menstrual period, the fourth week.

Advantages of the patch are similar to those of the birth control pill. The patch is most effective if changed on the same day of the week for three weeks in a row. Unlike the pill, which has to be taken daily, the patch needs to be replaced just once a week.

Disadvantages include those similar to the ones associated with the birth control pill, although more women complain of breast discomfort with the patch. In addition, skin irritation may occur around the patch, and there is a chance of it falling off. If the patch does come off, a woman should replace it with a new one. Like the pill, the patch does not protect against STDs.

Vaginal ring

The **vaginal ring**—or NuvaRing—approved in 2001, is a flexible ring inserted in the vagina close to the cervix to prevent pregnancy. The ring is implanted during the first five days of a woman's menstrual cycle and left in place for three weeks. During this time it releases progesterone and estrogen. The ring is taken out during the fourth week when the woman menstruates. After her period, a new ring is inserted.

The advantages of the vaginal ring are similar to those of the pill and the patch. In addition, a woman needs to change the ring just once a month. However, a woman cannot fit the vaginal ring herself; it must be fitted by a physician. It also provides no protection against STDs. Side effects are similar to those experienced by users of the pill and patch, although the possibility of vaginal irritation or infection is greater with the ring.

Depo-Provera and Lunelle

Hormonal contraceptive injections, developed in the 1960s, include **Depo-Provera** and **Lunelle.** Depo-Provera is an injection of progesterone given every three months to prevent pregnancy. **Lunelle** contains both estrogen and progesterone and is injected monthly. Most women experience fewer side effects on Lunelle than Depo-Provera, because they receive fewer hormones in the monthly Lunelle shot.

There are several advantages to injectable contraceptives in addition to the ones they share with the pill, the patch, and the vaginal ring. These contraceptives require little action on the part of the female. There are no estrogen side effects from Depo-Provera, and one trip to the doctor provides up to three months of contraception.

Disadvantages are similar to those of the other forms of contraception that rely on hormones, including no STD protection, and the need for repeated office visits. In addition, side effects of Depo-Provera may include menstrual irregularities, no menstrual bleeding after one year of use, and **infertility**—the inability to get pregnant—for up to one year. Fertility usually returns within two to three months with Lunelle.

Norplant
Norplant consists of six silicon capsules placed under the skin on the inside of the upper arm to prevent pregnancy. The implant gradually releases progesterone to prevent pregnancy for approximately five years. Norplant has to be inserted and removed by a physician. The procedure of inserting Norplant takes about 10–15 minutes and costs about $500–$750, which includes a medical examination and a pregnancy test. This costs an average of approximately $150 a year. Early removal is possible at the request of the woman.

Norplant, although effective in preventing pregnancy, is currently unavailable, due to a substantial drop in demand following well-publicized lawsuits and related complaints. Approximately one-half of the women using Norplant reported difficulty in removing the device. Side effects, in addition to those reported with other hormonal methods of birth control, included lengthened menstrual periods, spotting, or no bleeding at all. Additional side effects included headaches, weight gain, acne, breast tenderness, hair growth, and ovarian cysts. Other forms of contraceptive implants are available in other countries and may become more readily available in the United States.

INTRAUTERINE DEVICES
Although not commonly used by teens, intrauterine devices (IUDs) are small plastic or copper devices implanted in the uterus by a physician. Two IUDs—Copper T–380A, known as ParaGard, and Levonorgestral IUD, known as Mirena—were approved in 2000 and are currently available in the United States. ParaGard is effective for 12 years and Mirena is effective for five years.

How IUDs prevent pregnancy is not completely understood. Researchers believe they prevent **fertilization,** the fusion of the egg and sperm, change the uterine lining, and affect the movement of sperm and eggs. Mirena releases small amounts of progesterone. Both types of IUDs cost about $175–$500.

The advantages of IUDs include an effectiveness rate of over 95 percent. They also require little thought once implanted. The disadvantages include an increased risk of **pelvic inflammatory disease,** a bacterial infection that may result in scar tissue buildup in the **fallopian tubes,** and **ectopic pregnancy** (a pregnancy in which the fertilized egg implants in a fallopian tube instead of the uterus). The two fallopian tubes extend from each side of the uterus to the ovaries where fertilization takes place. Uterine cramps, backache, heavy menstrual flow and bleeding, and spotting may occur as a result of an ectopic pregnancy.

If a woman with an IUD becomes pregnant, there is a greater chance of a miscarriage. IUDs are not recommended for women who still plan to have children, due to an increased risk of infection and possible infertility.

BARRIER METHODS

Barrier methods physically block the sperm from reaching the egg. They are commonly used with **spermicides**–vaginal film, foams, creams, or gels. These substances, which can be purchased over the counter, contain a chemical that kills sperm. The most common barrier methods are condoms and the diaphragm.

Male condom

The male condom, the most common contraceptive used by teens, covers the penis during intercourse to collect semen and sperm. Condoms are effective if used correctly and used every time. Condoms made of latex work best, because they also protect against STDs and HIV. Condoms made of lambskin are not recommended, because they have pores and therefore do not protect against STDs and HIV, the virus that causes AIDS.

Condoms protect against STDs, are inexpensive, and do not require a prescription. They can be used during oral sex to protect the mouth against STDs. The most common complaints of condom users are that they interfere with spontaneity and diminish sensation. Only about one or two condoms in 100 break.

Q & A

Question: How do I put on a condom?

Answer: There are several important steps to using a condom correctly to prevent pregnancy or STDs. First, check the expiration date on the package to be sure the condom has not expired. When condoms get old they break more easily. Second, the package must have an air pocket. No air may be a sign that someone may have poked a hole in the package with a sharp object. As a result, the condom may have dried up. To test for an air pocket, gently pinch the package with a thumb and pointer finger.

Next, carefully open the package, making sure not to tear the condom with fingernails, teeth, or rings. The condom should be put on an erect, or hard, penis before it comes into contact with a partner's mouth, vagina, or anus. Unroll the condom about half an inch before putting it on the penis. The tip is designed to contain semen. Pinch it while putting on the condom to clear the air. Air trapped in the tip may cause the condom to break.

If the condom is not put on correctly or doesn't roll down, it must be thrown away. Don't flip it over and use it again. The underside of the condom may now have pre-ejaculatory fluid on it that contains sperm or an STD. Finally, unroll the condom to the base of the erect penis.

For extra lubrication, and to prevent breaking, lubricants like K-Y Jelly, water, or spermicides can be used. Never use oil-based products like lotion, oils, or petroleum jelly. These products break down the condom and can cause a yeast infection in women. After ejaculation, remove the condom while the penis is still erect to keep it from slipping off. Slowly roll the condom off. Never reuse a condom.

Female condom

The female condom is a plastic pouch that fits inside the vagina. The closed end has a ring that covers the cervix and catches semen; the open end stays outside the vagina, so that the penis can enter. Female condoms can be purchased at drugstores.

The advantages of female condoms are that they protect against STDs, are relatively inexpensive, and can be placed in the vagina up to eight hours before intercourse. The disadvantages are that they cannot be used with a male condom and may slip out of place. They also require that the woman be comfortable enough with her body to insert it correctly.

TEENS SPEAK

I Was Too Shy to Carry a Condom

I'm a 16-year-old girl who wondered, "Why should I have to carry a condom?" I used to think girls looked "ready" for sex if they carried a condom. I also felt it wasn't up to us.

That it was the guy's job. Now I think differently. I've been dating my boyfriend for over a year and thought he would always be prepared when the time came. I was wrong.

One night we decided to have sex. I asked if he had a condom and he said, "No." I was shocked. I just figured he'd be ready since he was the guy. I know now I shouldn't assume things like that. For all I know, he could have assumed I was on the pill. Since he didn't have a condom, we decided to wait. We knew the risks of having sex without one and decided to wait until we were prepared.

It's a two-way street, and both people are responsible. We now talk about all of our options for contraception to see what will work best for us. I feel so much better now that we've talked about it. I think it's brought us closer.

Diaphragm and cervical cap

The **diaphragm** is a dome-shaped rubber cap with a flexible rim placed deep inside the vagina to cover the cervix and collect semen. The diaphragm must be left in place for six to eight hours after intercourse to work properly. However, it should not be left in longer than 24 hours. A prescription is required to obtain a diaphragm, because a physician must measure the cervix for a perfect fit. The diaphragm should be replaced once a year, or when a woman gains or loses more than 10 pounds.

The advantages of the diaphragm include a high rate of effectiveness when used with a spermicidal cream or jelly and minimal side effects. The woman also has the option of inserting the diaphragm in the vagina up to two hours before intercourse. The disadvantages of this method include an increased risk of urinary or vaginal infections, messiness of use, the need to be comfortable with one's body, and no protection against STDs.

Although not as commonly used as the diaphragm, the **cervical cap,** a thimble-shaped rubber barrier, also fits snugly over the cervix to block semen. The cervical cap is smaller than a diaphragm and therefore may be more comfortable for some women. It can be worn for as long as 48 hours. However, more women report inflammation and infection of the cervix as well as difficulty with insertion and removal than with the diaphragm.

DID YOU KNOW?

Percentage of Teens Who Used Safe Contraceptives, 2007

Grade	Percentage who reported having sex in the past 3 months and using a condom during last intercourse	Percentage who reported having sex in the past 3 months and using birth control pills during last intercourse
Total	61.5	16.0
9	69.3	8.7
10	66.1	11.6
11	62.0	15.0
12	54.2	23.5

Source: Centers for Disease Control and Prevention, 2007.

STERILIZATION

Permanent methods of contraception are referred to as **sterilization.** Two permanent methods are tubal ligation and vasectomy. These surgeries are intended for people who have already had children or are certain they never want children.

Tubal ligation

Tubal ligation is the surgery for women in which the fallopian tubes are blocked to prevent fertilization. The fallopian tubes are cut and tied off to keep an egg from reaching the uterus or sperm from reaching an egg in the fallopian tubes. This surgery is commonly referred to as "getting one's tubes tied." Although a woman will still ovulate and menstruate after this procedure, her body will absorb the unfertilized egg released in the abdominal cavity.

The surgery takes about 20 minutes in the hospital and most women return home the same day.

Vasectomy

The **vasectomy** is a surgery for men in which the **vas deferens** are cut and tied. The vas deferens are long, thin, sperm-carrying tubes that begin at each testicle and end at the **urethra,** the passageway for urine and semen. A man can still **ejaculate** (expel semen from the body through the penis), but no sperm are present, since they cannot travel through the vas deferens to the urethra. The surgery takes approximately 15–30 minutes, and most men return home the same day. Sperm is likely to be present for several weeks after a vasectomy, so a backup method for pregnancy prevention is required during that time.

WEIGHING OPTIONS

With the many types of contraceptives available, individuals need to know their options and what works best for them. Most people must also consider cost, availability, and comfort level. It is a good idea to discuss options with a partner before becoming sexually active. Experts recommend methods that protect against both unwanted pregnancy and STDs.

See also: Conception, Pregnancy, and Childbirth; Contraceptives Involving Risk; Pregnancy, Prevention of; Relationships and Responsibilities

FURTHER READING

Hatcher, Robert A., Anita Nelson, and Miriam Zieman. *A Pocket Guide to Managing Contraception.* Tiger, Ga.: Bridging the Gap Communications, 2007.
Kaiser Family Foundation. "Substance Use and Sexual Health among Teens and Young Adults in the United States." Washington, D.C.: Henry J. Kaiser Family Foundation, 2002.
Planned Parenthood Federation of America. *All about Birth Control: A Complete Guide.* New York: Three Rivers Press, 1998.

■ DATING

Dating is when you spend time with someone to get to know him or her for the purpose of seeing whether a romantic relationship will work. Dating can affect one's overall well-being in either a positive or negative way, depending on the relationship. Characteristics of a positive relationship include feelings of trust, safety, closeness, and openness with the other person. These are the characteristics of a healthy relationship.

SAFE DATING

Safe dating involves knowing the person you are going out with. Before deciding to go on a date, spend time with the person around others to see how he or she interacts with your friends. Talk to him or her at school, on the phone, and get to know his or her friends. The more you know about a person before you begin dating, the better.

When you go out on a date, a few things will help make the experience safe. Teens should let their parents know with whom they are going and where they will be. They should also leave a number where they can be reached or should check in with their parents by calling periodically. Giving a friend this information can also be helpful in case of an emergency. Carrying a cell phone is a smart idea.

Teens begin dating at different times. Some are eager to date in middle school, while others show little interest in dating until college. Usually parents decide when their son or daughter is old enough to date. Some parents let their children date when they turn 13. Other parents may not let their children go on dates until they are 18. Parents often set an age for dating to make sure their teen is mature and wise enough to make good decisions while out alone with someone else.

Going on a date means two people who are attracted to each other spending time together doing something fun. Dating can involve seeing a movie, going to a concert, having lunch or dinner, or just hanging out.

Some teens prefer to **group date,** or go on a date with several other couples. They find spending time with other couples puts less pressure on a relationship. Some parents insist on group dates before they allow their teens to go on a date with just one person. They consider group dates safer.

The process of dating can seem complicated. One person has to ask the other out on a date, which may feel overwhelming. The person who does the asking may wonder if he or she will be turned down, or rejected.

What are the rules about who sets up the date? Traditionally the male asked the female out, but today females ask males out just as often. Once two people have agreed to go out, they need to find an activity that is enjoyable and comfortable for both of them.

Dating should never include forcing someone to do something he or she does not want to do. Whatever happens on a date should be a joint decision. Either person can pay for the date. Typically whoever does the asking offers to pay. Some couples, however, prefer that each person pays his or her own way. Others take turns paying for dates. Neither person should expect anything from the other just because he or she paid for the date or bought a present. Taking someone on a date never gives a person the right to have sex or force a person to do anything he or she does not want to do.

Going on a date together doesn't mean the couple will have intercourse. Some couples date for years and never have sex. Dating doesn't automatically lead to intercourse or give either person in the relationship the right to have sex with the other person.

Fact Or Fiction?

Staying with an abusive boyfriend or girlfriend is OK if the couple loves one another.

The Facts: If someone truly loves you, he or she is not abusive or aggressive toward you. People who are abusive usually have personal problems to work out. However, they tend to take out their problems on other people. Don't let one of those people be you!

If a teen is in an abusive relationship, he or she needs to get help. No one has the right to physically or emotionally hurt another person or speak cruelly to him or her. If a teen is scared and feels his or her partner is abusive, talking to a parent or another adult and getting their support is important.

THE IMPORTANCE OF COMMUNICATION

To maintain and even improve a dating relationship, couples should learn to send clear messages, listen to one another, and express anger in appropriate ways. By communicating effectively, a couple can build a relationship that will be meaningful and rewarding for both partners.

Sending clear messages

The first step is sending clear messages. By being clear and direct, people run less risk of being misunderstood or misinterpreted. Each partner knows where the other person is coming from and what he or she wants or does not want. Experts suggest using "I statements" when sending messages to a partner. Instead of saying "You make me mad when you show up late," one could say, "I worry about you when you're not on time." Saying, "I get angry when..." instead of saying "You make me upset" helps a person take ownership of and responsibility for his or her own feelings.

TEENS SPEAK

I Told My Boyfriend I Wanted to Break Up with Him

Breaking up is never easy. I knew it would be difficult. I just didn't want to be in a relationship any more. The breakup was so hard. Our families are close, and we have a lot of the same friends. I didn't want to lose them too. I decided my true friends would stay my friends no matter who I dated.

I decided to tell him when we got home from school. I knew this would be better than doing it at school where everyone would find out right away. I didn't want him to be embarrassed in front of our friends or feel like he had to explain everything.

I took responsibility for my own feelings. I told him I wasn't ready for a long-term relationship. I told him I still cared about him deeply and that he meant a lot to me, just not in a boyfriend way. I enjoyed our time together and made sure he knew that. Overall he took it pretty well. He appreciated me telling him at home. All things have an ending, but at least we are still friends. I don't think that will ever end.

Listening

The second step in effective communication is listening. It is the hardest thing for many people to do. They have a tendency to plan what they will say next instead of listening to what the other person has to say. To show one is listening, he or she should make eye contact with the speaker. One should also not interrupt the speaker or give feedback until the person has finished speaking. Even though one may not agree with what the speaker saying, letting him or her feel heard and appreciated is important. For many people, talking about their feelings can be difficult.

Expressing anger appropriately

Appropriately expressing anger is the third step. Some people become angry easily and do not know how to express their feelings in an appropriate way. To resolve problems or improve the relationship without hurting one another, experts suggest agreeing to disagree. They also recommend:

- Not allowing anger to build up. If something happens, discuss it as a couple.
- Agreeing on a time and place to work out disagreements. Let the person know what will be discussed before meeting.
- Addressing anger in specific ways without bringing up the past disagreements.
- Attacking the problem and not each other. Use "I statements" and let the person know he or she is appreciated at the same time.
- Trying to understand each other's point of view.
- Knowing when it is time to stop. Taking a break and returning to the issue later may be necessary if things are not getting resolved.
- Not holding grudges. Let things go once the disagreement has been resolved.

Q & A

Question: My girlfriend gets jealous a lot. Is this okay?

Answer: Jealousy in a relationship is not healthy. If both people trust each other, there is no need for jealousy. Although jealousy may seem harmless and even playful at first, it can lead to serious quarrels and even violence. Jealous people usually have low self–esteem.

FROM FRIENDSHIP TO INTIMACY

Many dating couples begin as friends. They get to know each other and become comfortable with one another before dating. Being friends first helps to develop **intimacy** and trust. Intimacy is more than physical closeness. It includes commitment, caring, and self-disclosure. A person can be intimate with family and friends as well as a dating partner.

Just as relationships differ, so do types of love. The love you feel for a friend is different than the love you feel for a boyfriend or girlfriend, a sister or brother, or the person you someday hope to marry. Different types of love may each have different levels of intimacy, passion, and commitment.

Psychologist Robert Sternberg defined the different types of love in an article in *Psychological Review*. According to Sternberg, a **friendship** places much importance on sharing closeness and trust. **Infatuation** involves one person being completely absorbed with desire for another. Feelings are intense. In **empty love** two people stay together because they feel they have to, such as for the sake of the children or for financial reasons. In **romantic love** the couple experiences closeness and lust, but not commitment. However, commitment may develop with time. **Fatuous love** is passionate but lacks closeness. **Companionate love** is friendly affection with deep attachment, while **consummate love** includes passion, intimacy, and commitment.

PRESSURE TO SCORE

Many teens may feel pressure from their peers to have sex. Others think that having sex will make them popular or cool. If someone has sex when he or she is not emotionally ready, feelings are likely to get hurt. Having sex with someone is a big step and it should not be taken lightly. A person who pressures a boyfriend or girlfriend to have sex risks hurting that person.

Some males put pressure on their friends to become sexually active. Boys who pressure others should keep in mind that sex is not a recreational sport and girls are not sexual objects. They are individuals with emotions, feelings, and values.

Having sex with multiple partners puts a teen at a greater risk of getting an STD, becoming pregnant, and hurting other people's feelings. Sex should happen when both partners are ready, not when their friends think they are.

Some people use the term *stud* to describe a boy who has multiple partners, yet consider girls who have multiple partners "sluts." This is an example of the **double standard.** A double standard suggests an activity is appropriate for one person but not another. Some people believe the double standard is disappearing. Knowing the risks of STDs and teen pregnancy, more teens are becoming less tolerant of those who have multiple sex partners, male or female.

Q & A

Question: Will having sex make me happy?

Answer: Some people think that having sex makes them happy. Many people with low self-esteem may believe that having sex with someone will make them feel good about themselves. Usually it only makes them feel worse. They may eventually realize that the person they had sex with only wanted them for sex. It may have felt good at the time to be wanted, but when it is over it can really hurt emotionally.

SEXUAL ABUSE DURING DATING

According to recent studies, you or someone you know is likely to have experienced abuse in a dating relationship. Abuse may be physical, psychological, emotional, or sexual.

Psychological and emotional abuse may include swearing, insulting a partner, embarrassing him or her, or making threats. Other examples include trying to control the activities of a boyfriend or girlfriend or isolating him or her from family and friends. Efforts to destroy a boyfriend or girlfriend's self-confidence and self-esteem is also an example of psychological and emotional abuse.

Physical abuse includes hitting, shoving, or slapping. It also includes the use of a weapon, such as a knife or gun, against a boyfriend or girlfriend. Although both teen boys and girls report being victims of physical abuse, the Youth Violence Prevention Resource Center reports that teenage boys are much more likely to use force to control their girlfriends, while girls are more likely to act violently in self-defense.

Sexual abuse refers to all forced or unwanted sexual activity or rape. It also includes coercing or pressure someone who is under the influence of drugs or alcohol to engage in sexual activity.

According to the Youth Violence Prevention Resource Center, it is difficult to get accurate information about the frequency of dating violence. Teens rarely report abusive relationships and the few studies that ask about it are rarely consistent. Some are interested only in sexual abuse, while others include questions about emotional and psychological abuse.

A 2005 survey by the Centers for Disease Control and Prevention found that approximately 9 percent of male and female high school students said that they had been hit, slapped, or physically harmed by a boyfriend or girlfriend in the previous year. Approximately 11 percent of females and 4 percent of males also reported that he or she had been forced to have sexual intercourse against his or her

DID YOU KNOW?

Physical Abuse by a Boyfriend or Girlfriend

Grade or gender	Percent of teens hit, slapped, or physically hurt on purpose by a boyfriend or girlfriend during the past 12 months
9	8.5
10	8.9
11	10.6
12	12.1
Males 9–12	11.0
Females 9–12	8.8
Total	9.9

Source: Centers for Disease Control and Prevention, 2007.

will. Many more teens reported emotional and psychological abuse in their dating relationships.

According to FBI statistics, 80 percent of all sexual assaults are **acquaintance or date rapes.** An acquaintance or date rape is a sexual assault by someone the victim knows.

Getting a medical exam immediately after a person has been raped is critical. The rapist could have an STD or another infection, cause a pregnancy, or physically damage the victim. Although the victim may feel like showering after being raped, it is the wrong thing to do. By showering, the evidence of the rape is washed away. Some people are reluctant to see a physician because they are not sure they want to press legal charges. Just because someone gets a medical exam after being raped does not mean he or she must press charges.

Forcing sexual activity on someone, such as unwanted touching, restraint, or intercourse, is wrong whether dating or not. Sometimes a person uses drugs or alcohol instead of force. Doing so is still rape or sexual assault, and it is still a crime. When a person is intoxicated, or drunk, he or she is unable to give consent. Without consent, any sexual activity is a sexual assault.

People must be clear about their sexual limits. If someone doesn't want sex, stating so clearly will help eliminate his or her partner's uncertainty. Setting limits in the relationship and talking about how far each person intends to go is necessary. If someone disregards those limits and pressures his or her partner, it may be time to find a new partner who is more respectful.

Dating can be a positive experience as long as couples communicate and are respectful of each other. Teens should always let someone else know where they are going and with whom they will be, whether on an individual or group date. Not all people start dating at the same time, and there is no specific age one should begin dating.

Whether a teen goes on only one date with a person or dates a person for a period of time, he or she should be respectful of that other person and never force him or her to do something. Teens do not have to give in to peer pressure and have sex just because they are dating. The more teens communicate with their partner, respect their partner, and respect themselves, the happier teens in relationships will be.

See also: Affection, Appropriate; Relationships and Responsibilities; Sexual Predators; Violence, Sexual

FURTHER READING

Buss, David. *The Dangerous Passion: Why Jealousy Is as Necessary as Love and Sex.* New York: Free Press, 2000.

Hendrick, Clyde, and Susan Hendrick. *Close Relationships: A Sourcebook.* Thousand Oaks, Calif.: Sage, 2000.

■ DIABETES AND PREGNANCY

A condition in which the body cannot use the sugars and starches it takes in as food to make energy, and the effects it has on a mother and her developing baby. With this, the body either makes too little insulin in the pancreas, which is known as type 1 diabetes, or cannot use the insulin it makes to change sugars and starches into energy, which is known as type 2 diabetes. Gestational diabetes is another form of the condition, which develops during pregnancy. Like other forms of diabetes, gestational diabetes affects the way your body uses sugar. The result may be dangerously high blood-sugar levels that can affect the mother and the baby.

WOMEN AND PREEXISTING DIABETES

According to the March of Dimes organization, about one in 100 women of childbearing age has type 1 or type 2 diabetes before pregnancy. Pregnancy is considered risky for women with diabetes because of the increased risk of miscarriage, stillbirth, and birth defects in their babies. A study by Kaiser Permanente's department of research and evaluation shows that there is a rising number of women who have diabetes before becoming pregnant. Researchers kept track of 175,249 women who gave birth in 11 Kaiser Permanente hospitals in Southern California between 1999 and 2005. The number of pregnant adult women with preexisting diabetes doubled between 1999 and 2005. The number of teens who had diabetes and gave birth increased five times over.

The authors of this study state that pre-pregnancy diabetes is more dangerous and potentially harder to treat than gestational diabetes. Preexisting diabetes is more likely to lead to miscarriages, stillbirths, and babies with birth defects because pregnant women may have

DID YOU KNOW?

Diabetes Rate in Adults by State, 2001
(Includes Gestational Diabetes)

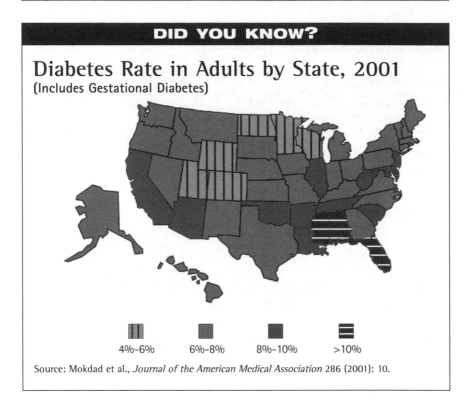

| 4%–6% | 6%–8% | 8%–10% | >10% |

Source: Mokdad et al., *Journal of the American Medical Association* 286 (2001): 10.

elevated blood sugar during the critical first trimester when the baby's organs are developing. However, provided they have good prenatal care and carefully monitor their blood sugar during pregnancy, most women with preexisting diabetes can look forward to healthy pregnancies and healthy babies.

Q & A

Question: Can a woman with diabetes before pregnancy prevent problems during the pregnancy for her and her baby?

Answer: If a woman with diabetes keeps her blood sugar in control before and during pregnancy, she can lessen her baby's risk of having a birth defect. Controlling the blood sugar also reduces the risk that a woman will develop common problems associated with diabetes, and reduce the risk that such problems will get worse during pregnancy. High blood sugar can lead to increased size in the baby. If a woman keeps her blood sugar in control, she can prevent this size and weight gain. This can be done through proper nurtitional habits, light exercise, and maintaining insulin injections if necessary.

GESTATIONAL DIABETES

When women develop diabetes because of their pregnancy it is known as gestational diabetes. Gestational diabetes is a type of diabetes that occurs only during pregnancy.

Causes and risk factors of gestational diabetes

It is not always known what causes gestational diabetes, but there are some indicators. During pregnancy, hormones or a shortage of insulin is often the cause of gestational diabetes.

During digestion, the body breaks down carbohydrates from foods such as bread, pasta, vegetables, fruits, and dairy products into various sugar molecules. One of these sugar molecules is **glucose,** a main source of energy. Glucose is absorbed directly into the bloodstream, but it can't enter the cells without the help of insulin. The pancreas, a gland located just behind the stomach, produces insulin continuously. When the blood sugar increases after eating, insulin production also increases. The extra insulin allows the cells to process more sugar, which provides the body with energy and helps maintain a normal level of sugar in the blood.

During pregnancy, the **placenta** produces hormones to sustain the pregnancy. Hormones from the placenta help the baby develop. These hormones also make cells more resistant to insulin. As the placenta grows larger in the second and third trimesters, it secretes more of these hormones, making it even harder for insulin to do its job. This problem is called **insulin resistance.** Insulin resistance makes it hard for the mother's body to use insulin. She may need up to three times as much insulin because of the resistance. Normally, the pancreas responds by producing enough extra insulin to overcome this resistance, but sometimes the pancreas can't keep up. When this happens, too little glucose gets into the mother's cells and too much stays in her blood. This is called **hyperglycemia.**

Although any woman may develop gestational diabetes, some of the factors that may increase risk are: a family history of diabetes, obesity, having given birth previously to a very large infant, a stillbirth or a child with a birth defect, and age (women who are older than 25 are at greater risk than younger women). Although increased glucose in the urine is often included in the list of risk factors, it is not believed to be a reliable indicator for gestational diabetes.

Gestational diabetes and the mother

Gestational diabetes usually develops during the second trimester—sometimes as early as the 20th week, but often not until later in the pregnancy. Gestational diabetes affects about 4 percent of all pregnant women—about 135,000 cases of gestational diabetes occur in the United States each year, according to the American Diabetes Association.

During pregnancy, it is best for women to have regular blood tests to check their blood-sugar level. These tests will let the doctor know if the woman's diet and exercise are keeping the blood-sugar level normal. If the woman's blood-sugar level is regularly high, the doctor may prescribe insulin to help lower it.

Fact Or Fiction?

Women can be screened for gestational diabetes.

The Facts: According to the American Pregnancy Association, approximately 2–5 percent of all expecting mothers will develop gestational diabetes. A screening for this disease usually will take place some time between the 24th and 28th week of pregnancy. Doctors test for gestational diabetes during this time because the placenta is producing large amounts of hormones that may cause insulin resistance. If the result comes back with elevated levels, further testing would be done to confirm a diagnosis of gestational diabetes.

Gestational diabetes and the baby

Gestational diabetes develops later in pregnancy, when the baby's organs are already formed. Because of this, gestational diabetes does not cause the kinds of birth defects sometimes seen in babies whose mothers had type 1 or type 2 diabetes before pregnancy. If her blood sugar is not controlled, a woman with gestational diabetes still has a greater chance of having a stillborn baby than a woman who doesn't have any form diabetes at all.

If the woman's blood sugar remains unregulated throughout the pregnancy, the baby likely will grow extra large. Unregulated diabetes causes the baby's blood sugar to be high. The baby makes more insulin and either uses the extra calories or stores them as fat. As a result, the baby is "overfed" and grows extra large. Extra large babies can occur in women with any diabetes—type 1, type 2, or gestational.

Other complications for the baby include low blood sugar, known as hypoglycemia. If a woman starts to breastfeed right away, the baby can get more glucose. If necessary, the baby may also need to get glucose through a tube into his or her blood.

The baby may also develop jaundice as a result of gestational diabetes. The baby's skin turns yellowish and the whites of the eyes may change color. This condition is easily treated and is not serious if treated properly. Babies born to mothers with gestational diabetes may also have low mineral levels in the blood. This problem can causes muscle twitching or cramping, but it can be treated by giving the baby extra minerals. In some cases, the baby may develop **respiratory distress syndrome**, where the baby has trouble breathing and needs oxygen or other help.

Can it be treated?

Gestational diabetes can hurt mothers and their babies. It is best to start treatment quickly. The treatment for gestational diabetes aims to keep blood glucose levels equal to those of pregnant women without the condition, which can include special meal planning and regularly scheduled physical activity. It is also important to be under the routine care of a doctor so that treatment can be monitored and changed if necessary.

Gestational diabetes usually goes away after pregnancy. But once a woman has had gestational diabetes, her chances are two in three that it will return in future pregnancies. In a few women, however, pregnancy even uncovers type 1 or type 2 diabetes. It is hard to tell whether these women develop gestational diabetes because they never knew they had diabetes or were treated for their type 1 or type 2 diabetes prior to becoming pregnant. The women would need to continue diabetes care depending on what type they have.

Many women who have gestational diabetes go on to develop type 2 diabetes years later. Gestational diabetes and type 2 diabetes both involve insulin resistance. Certain basic lifestyle changes may help prevent diabetes after gestational diabetes, such as losing weight, making healthy food choices, and exercising.

Women who have diabetes and want to have a baby should see a doctor before planning to conceive and establish good blood-sugar control. Women who have good blood-sugar control around the time of conception have no greater risk of having a baby with a birth defect than women without diabetes.

Q & A

Question: Will my baby have diabetes if I do?

Answer: Babies born to mothers with diabetes do not come into the world with diabetes. However, if the mother's diabetes was not controlled during pregnancy, the baby can very quickly develop low blood sugar after birth and must be watched very closely until his or her body adjusts the amount of insulin it makes. If the mother's diabetes is left untreated, this can lead to **macrosomia**, or a "fat" baby. Babies with macrosomia face health problems of their own, including damage to their shoulders during birth.

See also: Conception, Pregnancy, and Childbirth

FURTHER READING
American Diabetes Association. "Gestational Diabetes Resource Guide." Available online. URL: http://www.diabetes.org/gestational-diabetes.jsp. Accessed January 12, 2009.
American Pregnancy Association. "Gestational Diabetes." 2007. Available online. URL: http://www.americanpregnancy.org/pregnancy complications/gestationaldiabetes.html. Accessed January 12, 2009.
Centers for Disease Control and Prevention. "CDC Features: Diabetes & Pregnancy." Available online. URL: http://www.cdc.gov/Features/DiabetesPregnancy. Accessed January 12, 2009.

■ DRUGS, ALCOHOL, AND SEX

Drugs and alcohol are substances that are used to medicate or affect a person's mood. Mixing drugs and alcohol with sex can be risky.

The use of alcohol and other drugs often accompanies sexual inter-actions because many people believe that drugs enhance the sexual experience. In reality, drugs interfere with normal sexual function-ing. People tend to do things when they are under the influence of drugs or alcohol that they normally would not do. Both substances lower inhibitions, which may in turn lead people to risky sexual behaviors.

ALCOHOL AND SEX: THE "BEER GOGGLES"

People who drink are sometimes said to be wearing "beer goggles." They do not see things as clearly as they do when they are sober. Alcohol affects the parts of the brain that control judgment and inhi-bitions, which is why drinking may result in someone having risky sex or sex with no protection. Alcohol acts on the brain to reduce inhibitions of all kinds, including sexual ones. It is a depressant, and if the nervous system becomes too depressed, normal sexual responses are inhibited.

Fact Or Fiction?

Alcohol helps you perform better.

The Facts: Although alcohol may help a person feel more sociable, it does not enhance sexual performance. Alcohol can actually decrease a per-son's ability to perform sexually. A man may have difficulty getting and keeping an erection after drinking. A woman may have difficulty produc-ing lubrication. For both men and women, reaching orgasm may be more difficult under the influence of alcohol.

Being drunk at a party can lead to actions and feelings that one may regret the next day. Some people may regret having sex, while others may regret embarrassing themselves, hurting others, or hurt-ing themselves. Since alcohol affects judgment, an individual under the influence of alcohol does not think or act clearly.

To avoid potentially embarrassing situations, one should know how much he or she can safely consume. It does not take much alcohol to change how a person feels and acts. Even one drink can be too much.

TEENS SPEAK

I Learned the Hard Way

When I was 17 years old, I was at a friend's party and drank way too much. It was my first party, and I had no idea how much alcohol I could handle. I can barely remember some of the things I said and did that night. What I can remember is the ride home.

A guy I barely knew offered to give me a ride home. He ended up taking me to his house. His parents were out of town. He took advantage of me sexually. I was fading in and out of consciousness and said I didn't want him to touch me. He didn't listen, and I wasn't able to stop him. I think the only reason he didn't have sex with me is because I told him I was a virgin.

If he had tried to rape me, I wouldn't have been able to stop him. I was in a bad situation and was so scared. I hardly knew this guy and it was obvious he only wanted one thing. After that night I had nightmares and was depressed for a while. Now I know to take responsibility for myself and always stay in control. I don't drink much and always make sure I have a ride home. I never want to feel that way again. I also never want to be in a situation like that. I could have been raped!

DATE RAPE DRUGS

Date rape drugs are substances that reduce consciousness, memory, and the ability to properly function. Alcohol or drugs are involved in 90 percent of all rapes and sexual assaults, according to the Department of Justice in 2003. A sexual assault is any forced sexual activity. Rape—forced sexual intercourse—is a form of sexual assault.

Although alcohol is the most common date rape drug, a variety of others exist, including Rohypnol and gamma-hydroxybutyrate (GHB). Both are depressants that are colorless and odorless. Rohypnol comes in a pill form, and GHB is a liquid. Both are illegal. These drugs may cause a loss of consciousness and memory, drowsiness, slurred speech, blurred vision, breathing problems, and dizziness. They are even stronger when mixed with alcohol, since it too is a depressant.

Anyone who uses an illegal drug like Rohypnol or GHB for a sexual assault could face up to 20 years in jail and a fine of $250,000. Rape that involves these or similar drugs is known as **drug-facilitated rape**. To abide by the law, both parties must agree to have sex, but anyone who is drunk cannot legally give consent. Just because a person doesn't say no doesn't mean that he or she is saying yes. In some situations, such as being under the influence of drugs or alcohol, an individual may not be physically able to say no, even though he or she does not want sex. Others may be afraid to say no. They may fear violence if they refuse to have sex. Silence does not mean consent.

Rohypnol ("roofies")
Rohypnol is also known as roofies, roachies, Mexican Valium, and Roche. It is a pill that can easily be dissolved in a drink, which is why one should never leave a drink unattended. Rohypnol is said to be 10 times stronger than other depressants. Even just a small amount can make someone black out for up to 12 hours. When the person awakes, he or she may be unable to remember what happened. Some people may not be able to recall parts of the evening, and others forget everything that happened.

DID YOU KNOW?

Teen Sex and Alcohol or Drug Use

Grade in school	Percentage of teens who combined drugs or alcohol with sex in the previous three months
9	21.8
10	23.6
11	21.6
12	22.6
Total	22.5

Source: Centers for Disease Control and Prevention, 2007.

Q & A

Question: What do I do if I think my friend was slipped roofies?

Answer: If you think a friend was slipped roofies, take him or her to the hospital as quickly as possible. The drug remains in the body for 72 hours. At the hospital, a health-care professional will do a urine test to see if roofies are in the body. If Rohypnol is present, your friend may have been sexually assaulted, so the doctor will check for signs of an assault.

GHB

GHB is also called goop, gamma-on, and liquid ecstasy. Like roofies, it can result in unconsciousness and memory loss. When mixed with alcohol, it, too, becomes more dangerous. Some people take small amounts of GHB to increase the effects of alcohol. Taking GHB while drinking is risky, since one can never be certain of the drug's effect, especially when it is mixed with alcohol.

PROTECTING YOURSELF WHEN PARTYING

Partying can be fun but also risky. Experts suggest using these tips the next time you go to a party:

- Know your sexual limits and communicate them clearly. Don't give someone the wrong idea by acting sexually interested when you are not.
- Avoid alcohol. If you drink, know your limit. Stay in control and, most important, get out of a dangerous situation as quickly as possible.
- If you set a drink down or leave it unattended, throw it away.
- Never accept a drink from a stranger. Say, "I'd rather have a soda," "I'm the designated driver," or "Thanks, but I'm not drinking tonight."
- Always stay close to friends and travel in a group. Friends can help keep each other safe.
- Carry a cell phone, or know how to get to a phone if necessary.

■ Carry a few extra dollars in case money is needed to take a cab home.

DRUGS AND PREGNANCY

All drugs, including alcohol, affect the **fetus,** the developing baby. Whatever a pregnant woman puts into her body will have a greater impact on the fetus than on the woman. Doctors tell women to not even take aspirin when they are pregnant. The only drug doctors sometimes permit if absolutely necessary is acetaminophen in small amounts. Even over-the-counter cold medicines can be dangerous. Any legal or illegal drug can result in birth defects or other serious health problems for the baby.

Q & A

Question: Can my girlfriend smoke while she's pregnant?

Answer: Smoking while a woman is pregnant can lead to a low-birth-weight baby and other serious health problems. Smoking also increases a woman's chance of a miscarriage. Since smoking reduces the amount of oxygen in the blood, the baby's growth can be slowed down. Babies born to mothers who smoke are also at increased risk of a cleft lip and palate. Secondhand smoke is also dangerous. Infants who are around smokers are more likely to have breathing problems throughout their lives.

ALCOHOL AND PREGNANCY

During the first few months of pregnancy, the major organs of the fetus are forming. Alcohol can affect the development of those organs. **Fetal alcohol syndrome** (FAS) is a combination of birth defects in babies born to mothers who consume alcohol during pregnancy. These birth defects include mental retardation and retarded growth. Fetal alcohol syndrome is the third leading cause of birth defects among newborns. If a woman is trying to get pregnant or may think she is in the early stages of pregnancy, she should not drink. People may say, "One drink will not hurt the baby." Doctors don't know for sure, but they do know that alcohol, like everything else a woman puts in her body when she is pregnant, reaches the fetus.

THE IMPORTANCE OF BEING AWARE

Combining drugs or alcohol with sex can lead to risky behaviors. People tend to not think as clearly when they are drinking and engage in sexual behaviors that put them at a greater risk for an unwanted pregnancy or a sexually transmitted disease. By knowing one's limit and avoiding sex while under the influence of alcohol, a person can protect himself or herself from unwanted outcomes.

See also: Birth Defects and Risk-Taking Behaviors; Dating; Pregnancy, Prevention of; Relationships and Responsibilities; Sex and the Law; Violence, Sexual

FURTHER READING

National Institute on Drug Abuse. "NIDA InfoFacts: Club Drugs." National Institute on Drug Abuse Web site. Available online. URL: http://www.drugabuse.gov/Infofacts/clubdrugs.html. Accessed February 19, 2009.

Substance Abuse and Mental Health Services Administration (SAMHSA). *Drug Abuse Warning Network: Club Drugs, Update.* Rockville, Md.: SAMHSA, 2001.

U.S. Drug Enforcement Administration (DEA). *Drug Intelligence Brief: An Overview of Club Drugs.* Arlington, Va.: DEA, 2000.

■ FERTILITY

See: Conception, Pregnancy, and Childbirth

■ HEPATITIS

An inflammation of the liver caused by a virus. It can be caused by one of many things, including a bacterial or viral infection, liver injury caused by the ingestion of a toxin (poison), and even an attack on the liver by the body's own immune system.

The liver is an essential organ. It is as necessary to sustain life as is the heart. The liver is one of the body's powerhouses. It helps process nutrients and **metabolizes** medication. The liver also helps clear the body of toxic waste products, like those produced after breaking down food, alcohol, and even the insecticides used in treating some of the foods we eat.

Although there are several forms of hepatitis, in the United States the condition is usually caused by one of three viruses: the hepatitis A, hepatitis B, and hepatitis C viruses. Some hepatitis viruses can mutate, which means they can change over time and be difficult for the body to fight. In some cases, hepatitis B or C can destroy the liver. If this happens, the patient will need a liver transplant to survive, which is not always available or successful.

HEPATITIS A

The hepatitis A virus, or HAV, is found in the stool of persons with hepatitis A. It is usually spread by close personal contact or by consuming contaminated food or drinking water. The virus can also be spread by a combination of anal and oral sex. Good hygiene and proper sanitation can help prevent the spread of hepatitis A. There is also a hepatitis A vaccination.

Symptoms and treatment

Hepatitis A can cause mild flu-like illness, jaundice (yellowing of the skin), severe stomach pains, and diarrhea. According to the Centers for Disease Control and Prevention (CDC), people with hepatitis A often have to be hospitalized (up to about one person in five). Sometimes patients die as a result of hepatitis A (about three to five deaths per 1,000 cases). However, hepatitis A is considered to be less severe than the other forms of the virus. This is because hepatitis A rarely leads to permanent liver damage. Within a few weeks, the symptoms go away naturally, and the hepatitis A virus will no longer be in a person's system. Once someone has recovered from a hepatitis A infection, he or she has immunity to the virus, meaning that person will probably never get it again.

HEPATITIS B

The hepatitis B (HBV) virus can move from one person to another through blood and other bodily fluids. It can be transmitted through sexual intercourse and through needles, such as those shared by drug or steroid users or tattoo needles that haven't been properly sterilized. Because hepatitis B can be transmitted easily through blood and most body fluids, abstaining from sex or always using latex condoms if sexually active, avoiding contact with an infected person's blood, not using intravenous drugs or sharing any drug paraphernalia, and not sharing items like toothbrushes or razors can prevent hepatitis B infection.

To help prevent the spread of hepatitis B, health-care professionals wear gloves at all times when in contact with blood or body fluids. They are also usually required to be immunized against HBV. You cannot catch hepatitis B from an object someone has touched, such as a toilet seat.

Symptoms and treatment

Someone with hepatitis B may have symptoms similar to those caused by other viral infections, such as the flu. These include tiredness, nausea, loss of appetite, mild fever, and vomiting, as well as abdominal pain or pain underneath the right ribcage where the liver is. Hepatitis B can also cause jaundice and may cause the urine to appear brownish.

Symptoms may appear one to four months after someone has been exposed to hepatitis B. Some people with hepatitis B don't notice symptoms until they become quite severe. Others have few or no symptoms but are still able to transmit the disease. Some people's immune systems cannot fight the infection entirely and remain contagious for the rest of their lives.

Vaccination

There is an immunization (vaccine) against hepatitis B. The immunization is given as a series of three shots over a six-month period. Newborn babies in the United States now routinely receive this immunization series. Of babies born to women who have the hepatitis B virus, 90 percent will also have the virus unless they receive a special immune injection and the first dose of hepatitis B vaccine at birth. Teens who see their health-care provider for yearly exams are also likely to be given the hepatitis B immunization if they haven't had it before. According to the Society of Obstetricians and Gynecologists of Canada, immunization programs have been responsible for a significant drop in the number of cases of hepatitis B among Canadian teens over the past 10 years.

If someone has been recently exposed to the hepatitis B virus, a doctor may recommend a shot containing antibodies against the virus to try to prevent the person from coming down with the disease. For this reason, it's especially important to see a doctor quickly after any possible exposure to the virus.

HEPATITIS C

Like hepatitis B, hepatitis C can lead to cirrhosis or liver cancer. Also like hepatitis B, hepatitis C is transmitted from person to person through blood or other body fluids. Hepatitis C is the most serious type of hepatitis. It's now one of the most common reasons for liver transplants in adults. Every year, more than 320,000 people become infected with a form of hepatitis, and thousands of people in the United States die from the virus. Furthermore, there is no cure and no vaccine.

According to statistics compiled by the Nemours Foundation, about 4.1 million Americans currently have the hepatitis C virus. The sharing of drug paraphernalia, such as needles, is a common cause for the spread of the virus. Having unprotected sex with an infected person can also cause the spread of hepatitis C. Prior to 1900, many people were infected with hepatitis C due to unsanitary blood transfusions. The blood screening process and handling procedures have improved greatly since then to prevent the spread of hepatitis C during blood transfusions.

Fact Or Fiction?

Injecting drugs is one of the main ways people become infected with hepatitis.

The Facts: Intravenous drug use is a common way of becoming infected with both the hepatitis C virus and HIV. According to the CDC, 50 to 90 percent of HIV-infected injection drug users are also infected with hepatitis C. This is especially problematic because the hepatitis C virus is much more serious in persons who have HIV. The combination leads to liver damage more quickly. It is not known yet, however, whether coinfection with the hepatitis C virus makes HIV/AIDS progress faster.

Although hepatitis C medications are helpful to people with the disease, they are not always easy to take. Some medications involve many injections.

See also: Sexually Transmitted Diseases (STDs)

FURTHER READING
Hirsch, Larissa. "Hepatitis." Available online. URL: http://www. kidshealth.org/teen/infections/stds/hepatitis.html. Accessed January 12, 2009.

Horn, Lyle W. *Hepatitis. Deadly Diseases and Epidemics.* New York: Chelsea House, 2005.

■ MEDIA AND SEX, THE

The media—newspapers, magazines, radio, television, and the Internet—is a way for many people to learn about sexual behavior. In a 2006 report from the Kaiser Family Foundation, it was noted that in a typical day more than eight in 10 (83 percent) children under the age of six use screen media, or TV, with those children averaging about two hours a day. Media use increases with age, from 61 percent of babies one year or younger who watch screen media in a typical day, for an average of one hour and 20 minutes, to 90 percent of four- to six-year-olds, for an average of two hours and three minutes.

Not surprisingly, the media helps shape young people's attitudes toward sex. Yet the message the media sends is often mixed. At times the media depicts sexual relationships in a positive way by featuring the connection between two loving adults. At other times, sex is shown in negative ways—ways that hurt or degrade people.

The Kaiser Family Foundation also reported in 2005 that 70 percent of all TV programs, including all genres except children's, news, and sports, contained some form of sexual content. Only 14 percent of those programs contained content that included references to the risks and responsibilities associated with sexual activity.

The media also influences ideas about sexual identity and gender roles by creating **stereotypes** of males and females. A stereotype is a label or judgment about an individual based on the characteristics of a group. As a result, some people may feel that they have to act in a certain way.

Fact Or Fiction?

The media does not affect the way teens view their sexuality.

The Facts: The media strongly affects people's view of sexuality and what is sexy, even though they may not be aware of it. The media influences what people consider sexy in a man or woman. Some people think that what they watch on TV or see in magazines is similar to real life. Although the media can be a source of information, it is also designed for entertainment. Therefore, one shouldn't always consider what he or she sees in the media to be real.

SEXUALITY ON TV

Television is one of the most pervasive and influential forms of mass communication. It affects views of sexuality through references to dating, relationships, and sexual activity. It also influences ideas about what is normal and expected.

The Kaiser Family Foundation reports that a majority of parents say they are "very" concerned about the amount of sex (60 percent) and violence (53 percent) their children are exposed to on TV. After being read arguments on both sides of the issue, nearly two-thirds of parents (63 percent) say they favor new regulations to limit the amount of sex and violence on TV during the early evening hours, when children are most likely to be watching (35 percent are opposed).

Sexuality and sex on television can be explicit. Images range from flirting to sexual intercourse. In the 1950s, TV stations could not show a husband and wife sleeping in the same bed. Today, most of the sexual activity on TV involves unmarried couples, which may send a message that sex outside of marriage is acceptable, normal, or even expected.

The Kaiser Family Foundation conducts a study every two years to examine sexual messages on television. Their study of the 2004–05 season found that 70 percent of shows on TV included scenes with significant sexual contact, an increase from the 1997–98 season, in which about one-half of all TV shows included sexual contact. Additionally, only 14 percent of all shows with sexual contact mentioned potential risks associated with sexual activity, such as sexually transmitted diseases or unplanned pregnancy.

Portrayals that included sexual risks (STDs or becoming pregnant), abstinence, or the need for sexual safety were present in 15 percent of the shows with sexual content. Hence, sexual content on TV is more likely to promote sexual activity among American adolescents than it is to discourage it.

Not every program exploits sex. A number of talk shows address sensitive issues and educate the public by providing expert opinions on how to improve relationships and deal with rape and child abuse. TV can also educate people on same-sex relationships, varying lifestyles, and the characteristics of healthy relationships. Some people are reassured by programming that reveals that others have problems similar to their own.

THE IMPACT OF TV AND MOVIES

According to *Sex on TV 4*, a biennial study published by the Kaiser Family Foundation in 2005, the number of sexual scenes in TV has nearly doubled since 1998. Research confirms that, despite increases in the amount of time spent with video games and the Internet, TV continues to dominate young people's media use, with eight- to 18-year-olds watching an average of three hours a day. Three out of four 15- to 17-year-olds think sex on TV influences his or her own behavior.

A study conducted by the RAND Corporation took a sample of more than 1,700 12- to 17-year-olds and found that those who were heavy viewers of sexual content were twice as likely to initiate sexual intercourse over the next year as those who saw the least amount of sexual content.

The RAND study also found that for African-American youth, those who watched more TV shows that included storylines about safer sex, or the risks and responsibilities of sexual activity, were less likely to initiate intercourse in the next year.

- Adolescents reported that television is equally or more encouraging about having sex than their best friend.

- Female college students who frequently watched sexually suggestive music videos had more permissive attitudes about sex than did light viewers.

- Adolescents who were shown a set of 10 music videos were more likely to find premarital sex acceptable than a comparison group who did not see the videos.

The *Sex For TV 4* study conducted by the Kaiser Family Foundation also found that in 2004–05, 70 percent of the total week sample of nearly 1,000 programs included some sexual content, either talk about sex or portrayals of sexual behavior. The programs that contained sexual content averaged five scenes per hour that involved sexual themes or topics. This means that the base of TV programs that convey sexual messages has increased by exactly 25 percent, while at the same time the number of scenes with sexual topics in those shows has risen 5 percent since 1997–98.

According to the survey, whether they want it or not, children and teens are constantly being exposed to sexual imagery. The average American teen watches three to four hours of television every day and for every hour of television he or she watches, there are, on average, 6.7 scenes including sexual topics, about 11 percent of which show couples engaged in sexual intercourse. Similar sexual content can be found on teen-oriented radio, CDs, and the Internet.

Q & A

Question: How can I become more aware of the way the media uses sexual images?

Answer: Experts suggest that asking yourself the following questions can be helpful in critical viewing:

- Who has created the sexual images?
- Who is engaging in the sexual behavior?
- From whose perspective does the camera frame events?
- Whose viewpoint is not heard?
- How would your parents, girlfriend, or boyfriend talk about the story you just saw?
- What is your role as a spectator in identifying with, or questioning, what you see and hear?
- Who owns the medium? How much do the owners profit from showing sexual content?

SEXUALITY IN ADVERTISING

Advertisers use sex to sell everything from cars and furniture to cosmetics and clothing. Beautiful, strong, or sexy people are often used to promote a broad range of products. The average person doesn't necessarily look like the models used in advertising. People see hundreds of ads per day, either on clothing, billboards, commercials, or in magazines.

Sexuality in advertising can be negative because it tends to desensitize people to behaviors that are considered unacceptable in most situations. If people see a behavior over and over again, they may begin to accept what they see even though they know it is illegal or harmful. For example, some ads use forms of sexual aggression to sell products. Media experts encourage viewers to study ads closely and question what advertisers are portraying.

Magazines often contain articles that promise to reveal "how to be sexy" or "how to have the best sex ever." These articles often tap into people's insecurities. The ads may make people think they need to be sexier or more attractive. Those who tend to be insecure about their looks or their relationships may buy the magazine just for the "how-to" article. According to the 2002 book, *Sexual Teens, Sexual Media*, the majority of editorial content and advertising in magazines such as *Seventeen* and *Glamour* remain focused on what girls and women should do to get and keep their man, even though over the past decade, these magazines have also increased their coverage of sexual health issues.

PORNOGRAPHY

Pornography is creative activity of no literary or artistic value other than to stimulate sexual desire and arousal. Pornography can range from two consenting adults in sexual activity to nudity and stripping. Some even show criminal acts such as rape and other forms of sexual assault. Pornography is currently a multibillion dollar industry. It can be found in a variety of media, including TV, magazines, videos, and the Internet.

Pornography can be dangerous, particularly if it exploits children or teens. Pornography that includes people under the age of 18 is illegal throughout the nation. It is never acceptable to involve children or teens in pornography. Although scholars disagree on the effects of pornography on adults, they generally agree it has a negative effect on young people.

SEXUALITY ON THE INTERNET

As of 2008, 73.6 percent of all adults in the United States had Internet access, according to 2008 World Internet Usage Statistics. By 2012, it is expected that 90 percent will have access to broadband services. Some Internet sites provide accurate information regarding relationships or sexual health. However, others show sexuality in a negative way by displaying pornography.

Many people visit sexuality-related Web sites daily. These sites range from chat rooms for people with sexually transmitted diseases or AIDS to wig-care tips for transsexuals. In 2006, an online victimization report noted that one in 11 of 10- to 17-year-olds who are regular Internet users encountered unwanted pornography in the past year. One in seven teens had been exposed to unwanted sexual solicitations or approaches. At the same time, many sites, including the American School Health Association's www.iwannaknow.org, promote healthy sexual behavior and provide answers to questions regarding sexuality.

Cybersex, sexual arousal as a result of images or words on a computer, may involve fantasizing, talking about sex, or **masturbating** (stimulating the genitals for pleasure). On the Internet, one can find interactive adult bookstores that present products and live "cyberstrippers." One can view live video containing sexual acts and become involved in interactive sexual talks.

Most of these Internet browsers use cybersex as a way to "experience" sex. Some users, however, perhaps 8 to 10 percent, become hooked on cybersex and may experience significant life problems as a result. A variety of consequences can result from heavy use of cybersex, including isolation, neglect of family life, loss of job, and emotional and health risks.

A **pedophile** is a molester of children or teens. Pedophiles may have other online friends who exchange child pornography and discuss experiences with molesting children. They cruise chat rooms for children and teens and gain their trust by pretending to be friendly and caring. Then, the pedophile tries to get children and teens to agree to e-mail with them or talk on the phone. It is important to not trust people on the Internet since they can pretend to be anyone. You can never be sure who you are really talking to.

Those who enjoy taking part in discussions on Internet chat rooms can protect themselves from pedophiles and other dangerous individuals by taking a few precautions. If someone in a chat room asks a question that is too personal, leave that conversation. Questions like, "What are you wearing?" or "Can we meet later?" may suggest that the questioner is dangerous. The conversation should be ended if anyone gets too personal or makes you feel uncomfortable.

If you think you are speaking with someone on the Web who may be dangerous, inform a trusted adult. Do not continue to communicate with a potentially dangerous person online or in person. If the individual is persistent, he or she may become a threat, and it may become necessary to involve the police.

In an emergency, a teen feeling unsafe or uncomfortable could also pretend to be a parent online and threaten to call the police if this person doesn't leave "your son or daughter" alone. This may scare them enough to end their efforts in communication, but the incident should still be reported to an adult.

MEDIA TODAY

Sexuality is commonly found in all media. The media suggests how one should look, what products to buy, and what is considered normal for men and women. Sexual behavior can be found on TV, in magazines, in advertisements, on billboards, and on the Internet. The media's main purpose is entertainment and advertising. Knowing this, people can more easily remember that much of the media, other than news and educational programs, is not always reality.

See also: Sexual Predators

FURTHER READING
Brown, Jane D., Jeanne R. Steele, and Kim Walsh-Childers, eds. *Investigating Media's Influence on Adolescent Sexuality.* Mahwah, N.J.: Lawrence Erlbaum, 2001.
Hawk, Skyler, et al. "Adolescents' Contact with Sexuality in Mainstream Media." *The Journal of Sex Research* 43, no. 4 (2006).

■ PELVIC INFLAMMATORY DISEASE

A serious infection that affects the reproductive organs of a female. PID usually occurs when sexually transmitted bacteria spread from the vagina to the uterus and upper genital tract. PID can result in infertility or complications during pregnancy.

Pelvic inflammatory disease is an infection in the female reproductive organs (**uterus, fallopian tubes,** and **ovaries**). Normally, the **cervix** (opening to the womb) prevents bacteria in the **vagina** from spreading up into the uterus, fallopian tubes and ovaries. However, if the cervix is exposed to a sexually transmitted disease (STD) such as **gonorrhea** or **chlamydia**, which are caused by bacteria, it becomes infected and allows bacteria to pass through. If this occurs, the woman's fallopian tubes may be damaged by the spreading bacteria, making it difficult for her to become pregnant.

Although the bacteria that causes PID most commonly spread through sex, they may also enter the body after gynecological procedures such as the insertion of an intrauterine device (IUD) (a form of contraception), childbirth, and miscarriage. Oral contraceptives ("the pill") are thought, in some cases, to enhance cervical ectropion, a condition that allows easier access to tissue where bacteria may thrive. However, oral contraceptives may, in other cases, have a protective role against developing PID because they stimulate the body to produce a thicker cervical mucus, which is harder for semen (which may contain bacteria) to penetrate. This makes it more difficult for semen to transmit bacteria to the uterus.

Also, during most of a woman's menstrual cycle, the cervical mucus at the opening of the cervix is thick and acts like a plug, keeping sperm and bacteria from entering the uterus. The plug dissipates during ovulation (when rising levels of estrogen make the mucus clear, thin, and watery) and menstruation, making it easier for bacteria to enter the uterus and upper reproductive tract. Sometimes during menstruation, many women experience backward menstrual flow, or retrograde menstruation. The backward flow can carry microorganisms as it moves back from the uterus to the fallopian tubes.

According to the National Institutes of Health, nearly 1 million U.S. women develop PID each year. Women between ages 15 and 25 have the highest incidence of PID. It is estimated that one in eight sexually active adolescent girls will develop PID before reaching age 20. Women can protect themselves from PID by taking action to prevent STDs or by getting early treatment if they do get an STD.

WHAT TO WATCH FOR

Because PID is frequently undiagnosed, statistics are probably greatly underestimated. Risk factors include sexual activity during adolescence, multiple sexual partners, past history of PID, and past history of any sexually transmitted disease. Some of the typical symptoms of someone suffering from pelvic inflammatory disease include dull pain or tenderness in the lower abdomen, burning or pain when you urinate, nausea and vomiting, bleeding between menstrual periods, increased or changed vaginal discharge, pain during sex, and fever and chills. It is possible for a woman to have PID and be without symptoms, or have symptoms too mild to notice, for an extended period of time.

Upon the start of treatment, the symptoms may go away before the infection is cured. Even if symptoms go away, the woman should finish taking all of the prescribed medicine. This will help prevent the infection from returning.

COMPLICATIONS

PID can be cured with several types of antibiotics. The longer a woman delays treatment for PID, the more likely she is to become infertile or to have a future **ectopic pregnancy** because of damage to the fallopian tubes.

Early and complete treatment can help prevent complications of PID. If PID isn't treated, it can cause permanent damage to your internal organs. Scar tissue can form in the fallopian tubes and around the abdomen. This tissue can prevent pregnancy or cause the pregnancy to form outside the uterus (called a tubal or ectopic pregnancy). Scarring can cause pain that lasts for months or even years. Occasionally, the effects of PID can be so severe that surgery is required to remove pus, get rid of scar tissue, or remove damaged organs.

Untreated PID also puts a woman at risk for a **tubo-ovarian abscess** (TOA). A TOA is a collection of bacteria, pus, and fluid that occurs in the fallopian tube. It is most often seen in teens. A TOA is also more likely to occur in teens or adult women who use intrauterine devices (IUDs) as birth control. A teen girl with a TOA often looks sick and has a fever and pain that makes it difficult to walk. The abscess can be treated in the hospital with antibiotics. Surgery may also be needed to remove it.

PID is more likely to come back if a woman is exposed to STDs again. Each instance of PID causes more damage and a greater possibility of complications.

Ectopic pregnancies

Ectopic means "out of place." In an ectopic pregnancy, a fertilized egg has implanted outside the uterus. The egg settles in the fallopian tubes in more than 95 percent of ectopic pregnancies. This is why ectopic pregnancies are commonly called tubal pregnancies. The egg can also implant in the ovary, abdomen, or the cervix, so you may see these referred to as cervical or abdominal pregnancies. A large proportion of the ectopic pregnancies occurring every year are due to the consequences of PID.

Infertility

Infertility is when a woman is not able to have children. In the United States, PID is the leading cause of infertility in women. Around 15 percent of those affected by PID have secondary infertility as a result—more than 100,000 women each year. Abscesses may form in the uterus, ovaries, and fallopian tubes. The infection causes scarring, which keeps the egg from traveling down the tubes, preventing pregnancy. The womb lining can also be so damaged that a potential embryo cannot implant.

DIAGNOSIS

The diagnosis of PID can be made when all three of the following symptoms are found during a pelvic exam: lower abdominal tenderness, tenderness of fallopian tubes and ovaries, and tenderness of the cervix. All other explanations for these findings must have been ruled out, so the healthcare provider may also order tests to identify the organism that led to the infection (such as chlamydia or gonorrhea) or to distinguish between PID and other problems with similar symptoms.

A pelvic ultrasound is a helpful procedure for diagnosing PID. An ultrasound can view the pelvic area to see whether the fallopian tubes are enlarged or whether an abscess (pus-filled area) is present. In some cases, a **laparoscopy** may be necessary to confirm the diagnosis. A laparoscopy is a surgical procedure in which a thin, flexible tube with a lighted end (laparoscope) is inserted through a small incision in the lower abdomen. This procedure enables the doctor to view the internal pelvic organs and take specimens for laboratory studies, if needed.

Doctors diagnose pelvic inflammatory disease based on signs and symptoms, a pelvic exam, an analysis of vaginal discharge and cervical cultures. During the pelvic exam, the doctor uses a cotton swab to take samples from the vagina and cervix. The samples are sent to a laboratory for analysis to determine which organism is causing the infection. To confirm the diagnosis or to determine how widespread the infection is, the doctor may advise further testing to fully determine the diagnosis.

Fact Or Fiction?

The most common preventable cause of infertility is Pelvic Inflammatory Disease.

The Facts: PID is preventable through regular checkups and through early detection of STDs. The scarring that results from pelvic inflammatory disease (PID) can lead to infertility, tubal pregnancy, chronic pelvic pain, abscesses, and other serious health problems in women. PID is the most common preventable cause of infertility in the United States. Having sexual intercourse with only one partner and using contraceptives such as condoms with spermicidal lubricants reduces the risk of infection as well.

KEEPING YOURSELF SAFE

Because of the difficulty in identifying organisms infecting the internal reproductive organs, and because more than one organism may be responsible for an episode of PID, PID is usually treated with at least two antibiotics that are effective against a wide range of infectious agents. A healthcare provider will determine and prescribe the best therapy. However, antibiotic treatment does not reverse any damage that has already occurred to the reproductive organs. If a woman has pelvic pain and other symptoms of PID, it is critical that she seek care immediately. Prompt antibiotic treatment can prevent severe damage. If you have PID, further infection is common. After a first episode of PID, 20 percent of women have further episodes, mostly within two years.

Women being treated for PID should be reevaluated by their healthcare provider two to three days after starting treatment to be sure the antibiotics are working to cure the infection. In addition, a woman's sex partner(s) should be treated to decrease the risk of reinfection, even if the partner(s) has no symptoms. Although sex partners may have no symptoms, they may still be infected with the organisms that can cause PID and could transfer the infection back.

FURTHER READING

American Social Health Association. "Learn About STDs/STIs." Available online. URL: http://www.ashastd.org/learn/learn_pid.cfm. Accessed January 12, 2009.

Mayo Clinic Staff. "Pelvic inflammatory disease." Available online. URL: http://www.mayoclinic.com/health/pelvic-inflammatory-disease/DS00402. Accessed January 12, 2009.

■ PREGNANCY, PREVENTION OF

The period of time after conception during which a baby develops in the uterus. Preventing pregnancies implies forestalling conception—the fusion of the egg and sperm. If couples choose a method that is reliable and use it every time they have sex, prevention of conception is possible. Some of these methods protect only against pregnancy, but some also protect against **sexually transmitted diseases** (STDs). STDs are diseases that are spread through sexual contact.

ABSTINENCE

The only foolproof way to prevent pregnancy is **abstinence**—the conscious decision not to have sexual intercourse. It is a choice that a person can make at any time. Abstinence is 100 percent effective in preventing pregnancy.

Every time a couple has vaginal intercourse they are at risk of becoming pregnant. All three types of sex—vaginal, anal, or oral—put a person at risk for STDs. To be truly abstinent, two people do not share bodily fluids, including blood, **semen** (the ejaculated fluid containing sperm), and vaginal secretions. Couples who are abstinent from sexual intercourse may kiss, hug, and touch each other.

Relationships that involve sexual intercourse are filled with physical, emotional, and psychological risks. Abstinence provides teenagers the opportunity to avoid those risks. If it seems like everybody else is having sex, some people may feel they have to do it too, just to be accepted. The truth is that most teens are not having sex. A couple can still have a relationship without having sex. A decision made to not have sex is an important personal choice.

Abstinence is widely practiced. You do not have to be a virgin to practice abstinence. Sometimes people who have been having sex decide not to continue having sex. Abstinence is always available and free. It is easy to use as long as there is little or no pressure to have sex. Being assertive and standing up for one's beliefs makes it easier to be abstinent. Those who choose to be abstinent often increase their self-esteem, because they have made a decision and stuck with it. In addition, abstinence can strengthen a relationship. A mutual decision with a partner can bring a couple closer by talking about a sensitive, important topic.

Q & A

Question: How do I practice abstinence?

Answer: Although many people assume it is easy to be abstinent, it can be difficult in practice. The following tips can make abstinence a little easier.

- Decide in advance that you want to be abstinent and that it's your choice to make.
- Decide with your partner what activities you will say "no" to and what activities you will agree to. Make this decision consciously, ahead of time.
- Discuss other activities you and your partner might enjoy. These could include holding hands, massaging, dancing, kissing, or masturbating.
- Avoid situations that put pressure on you. To make abstinence easier, stay sober, stay aware—and stay out of the bedroom.
- Learn to say "no" and mean it. You have that right and responsibility. You don't have to give a reason—you can just say "No" or "I do not want to have sex."

WITHDRAWAL

Some people practice **withdrawal** to prevent pregnancy. The man withdraws his penis from a woman's **vagina** just before **ejaculation,** the process by which semen is forcefully expelled from the penis. If withdrawal is the only method a couple uses to prevent pregnancy, they are at risk of an unwanted pregnancy.

Withdrawal is not effective for two reasons. First, withdrawal relies on the male to control his ejaculation. Few men, especially younger men who can't always tell when they are going to ejaculate, have the level of control required. Men at all ages get so caught up in the heat of the moment that they usually can't stop.

Second, if a couple has sex a second time after using only withdrawal the first time, they increase their risk of getting pregnant. After ejaculating, **sperm** may be left in the male's **urethra,** or urinary tract through which both sperm and urine pass out of the body. Sperm is the male sex cell necessary for reproduction. However, sperm and urine never pass at the same time.

A male using the withdrawal method alone must urinate after having sex the first time before having sex a second time to clear any leftover sperm in the urethra. However, one can never be sure there is no sperm in the urethra. Leftover sperm may later come out in **pre-ejaculatory fluid,** or pre-cum, when the couple has sex again. This fluid is released from the penis during arousal and prior to ejaculation to lubricate the vagina. Furthermore, using the withdrawal method never protects people from STDs.

OUTERCOURSE

Practicing **outercourse** means a couple is sexually intimate by rubbing against each other, but no penetration occurs. Outercourse prevents pregnancy, as long as semen, which contains sperm, does not come near the vaginal opening. If a male ejaculates near the vaginal opening, his sperm can still enter the vagina and cause pregnancy. This form of pregnancy prevention does not protect from STDs.

RHYTHM METHOD

Some couples try to prevent pregnancy by using the **rhythm method.** They avoid intercourse on the days the woman is most likely to ovulate. **Ovulation** is a female's monthly release of an egg. Many women ovulate on day 14 of their cycle, with day one being the first day of their menstrual period. Since sperm can live in the woman's body for up to three days, couples who use the rhythm method should avoid sex from day 10 or 11 to day 17 or 18. This method is not reliable for females who do not have a regular **menstrual cycle,** including many teenage girls. A menstrual cycle is the hormonal interactions that prepare a woman's body for possible pregnancy. Ovulation is unpredictable.

CONTRACEPTIVES

Many couples use **contraceptives**—drugs, devices, or chemical agents that prevent pregnancy. Contraceptives include **hormonal methods,** such as birth control pills which prevent ovulation, and **barrier methods,** such as condoms and the diaphragm to block the sperm from meeting an egg.

The **birth control pill,** a hormonal method of contraception, is the most common form of birth control in the United States. The pill works by artificially changing **hormone** levels in a woman's body. A hormone is a chemical substance in the body that regulates the activity of other organs or cells. In this case, the hormones involved are **estrogen,** which regulates reproductive functions, and **progesterone,** which regulates the menstrual cycle and sustains pregnancy. The pill uses the two hormones or progesterone alone to prevent ovulation by changing the mucus lining of the **cervix**—the opening to the uterus—in order to block the passage of sperm or prevent the fertilized egg from implanting in the uterus.

Barrier methods of contraception physically block sperm from reaching an egg. Barrier methods include **condoms** and the **diaphragm.** A condom is a soft sheath of latex that fits over the erect penis to collect sperm. A diaphragm is a rubber cap with a flexible rim placed deep inside the vagina to keep sperm from entering the uterus. **Spermicides**—including foam, suppositories, creams and jellies—are commonly used in combination with the barrier methods. Spermicides contain a chemical that kills sperm.

PREVENTING AN UNWANTED PREGNANCY

Couples use a variety of ways to prevent pregnancy. Abstinence is the only foolproof method. For those who are sexually active, selecting a contraceptive method acceptable to both partners is important. Some also protect against STDs.

See also: Contraceptives Involving Risk; Contraceptives: Practices Proven Safe

FURTHER READING

Hatcher, Robert, Anita Nelson, and Miriam Zieman. *A Pocket Guide to Managing Contraception.* Tiger, Ga.: Bridging the Gap Communications, 2007.

Tone, Andrea. *Devices and Desires: Men, Women, and the Commercialization of Contraception in the United States.* New York: Hill and Wang, 2002.

■ PREGNANCY AND CHILDBIRTH, THE COST OF

The cost of pregnancy—the period of time in which a baby develops in the uterus—and childbirth can be quite high. No two women react to their pregnancy in the same way. Some are excited and happy, others may be fearful, and still others sad. But one thing that they all have in common is usually a realization that the financial and personal costs of having a baby are greater than they expected.

FINANCIAL COSTS OF HAVING A BABY

According to a recent study by the U.S. Department of Agriculture (USDA), it costs a middle-income family $250,000 to raise a child from birth to age 17, and that does not include the cost of a college education. In the first year alone, the costs of a baby can reach between $9,000 and $11,000, and most new and expectant parents do not realize the extent of the financial burden they are taking on.

The costs of having a baby include **prenatal care**—care to the expectant mother and fetus during pregnancy—and the costs of delivering the baby. For women who are covered by health insurance, most of these costs are covered. Women under age 18 may still be included on their parents' health insurance plan. Women who have no health insurance may have to pay the costs themselves or seek financial aid from such programs as **Medicaid,** a federal and state-funded program that provides assistance with medical costs for some low-income families and individuals.

Prenatal care and high-risk pregnancies

During pregnancy, many women choose to see an **obstetrician/ gynecologist** (ob-gyn). An obstetrician is a physician who treats pregnant women and delivers babies. A gynecologist diagnoses and treats disorders related to the female reproductive system. Other pregnant women may prefer to use a family doctor or a **midwife,** a registered nurse with additional training in child delivery.

Prenatal care costs can range from several hundred to several thousand dollars. Included in these figures are checkups for the pregnant woman and tests on her unborn child. Doctors test the expectant mother for sexually transmitted diseases (STDs) and check her weight and blood pressure.

Most pregnant women receive a **sonogram,** which is an image produced by the reflection of high-frequency sound waves, to observe the growth of the **fetus** (the developing baby). A sonogram can help the physician determine the age of the fetus, its growth pattern, position, and any abnormalities. If a physician sees signs of a problem, he or she may call for additional tests.

Most pregnancies have a healthy outcome. Some are complicated by problems with the expectant mother's health, the health of the fetus, or complications unique to the pregnancy itself. These complications result in 70-80 percent of the illnesses related to pregnancy by the mother and/or her child.

Complicated pregnancies require special prenatal care that can be extraordinarily expensive, but studies suggest that the money is well spent. The Institute of Medicine estimates that for every dollar spent on prenatal care, $3.38 could be saved in medical costs for low-birth-weight babies.

Many women choose to contact their local health department to find out about free or reduced-cost prenatal care since it is very expensive.

Delivery costs and more

Giving birth to a healthy baby in most communities across the nation involves a number of expenses. The costs usually include care during labor and delivery, a hospital stay (usually of one to three nights) professional and laboratory fees, and nursing costs for the infant and mother. A typical **vaginal birth**—the delivery of the baby through the **vagina,** the female organ known as the birth canal—costs approximately $6,000 to $8,000. According to the American Medical Association, approximately 70 percent of all deliveries are vaginal births.

If the baby has a dropping pulse, is positioned wrong, or is too big, a physician may perform a **cesarean section,** which is a surgical procedure in which a physician makes an incision through the abdominal wall and uterus to deliver the baby and **placenta.** The placenta is the structure through which the mother and fetus exchange materials such as nutrients and oxygen. The average cost of a cesarean delivery is approximately $10,000 to $12,000.

A cesarean delivery is more expensive because it is considered a major surgery and requires a longer stay in the hospital. During this time, both the mother and baby are checked and monitored regularly. According to the American Medical Association, about 30.3 percent of all deliveries are performed by cesarean section.

Delivery costs for more complicated births are much higher. Every year, nearly 4 million babies are born in the United States. Approximately 9.9 percent are low-birth-weight babies (less than 5.5 pounds), 1.3 percent are very low-birth-weight babies (less than 3.3 pounds), and more than 14.3 percent are preterm babies—babies that are born before the 37th week of pregnancy. These babies are not only "at risk" for a variety of medical problems but also place their parents at a significant financial risk.

Delivery costs for complicated births range from $20,000 to $400,000 per baby. According to the Pennsylvania Health Care Cost Council, premature babies represented 8.2 percent of all births in the state in 2002. The hospital charges for those babies represented one-half of all costs for newborn care—$600 million of the state's $1.2 billion in hospital costs. Costs in other states are similar.

Q & A

Question: If a couple is not married, is the father responsible for paying for the costs of having a baby?

Answer: Although the laws in each state may differ slightly, the father is usually financially responsible for child support. The amount of money he is required to pay is based on his salary. If the father is under age 18, his parents may be responsible for paying for the support of their son's child. Some males openly admit being the father and others do not, requiring the courts to determine fatherhood. Some males may not know for sure if they are the father. If a male is not sure if he is the father, he can ask for a blood test to find out.

THE FINANCIAL COSTS OF POSTNATAL CARE

Unless a mother decides to **breast-feed** her baby, one of the most expensive items an infant will need immediately is food. Mothers who breast-feed give their babies breast milk rather than a formula. If a mother decides to bottle-feed her child, a one-pound container of formula can be purchased for approximately $20. This amount of formula may last a week while the infant is still young. Eventually, a baby will require more than one can of formula a week. Formula alone could cost $80 to $100 dollars a month.

A program known as WIC is available to women as well. WIC, the Special Supplemental Nutrition Program for Women, Infants, and Children, provides nutritious foods, nutrition education, and referrals to health and other social services to participants at no charge. WIC serves low-income pregnant, postpartum, and breast-feeding women, and infants and children up to age five who are at nutrition risk. According to the USDA, more than 8 million people get WIC benefits each month.

Breast-feeding is a cheaper, healthier way to feed a baby. Breast milk is free, readily available, and healthier than formula. Breast milk contains **antibodies**—substances that fight infection in the body. Children who are breast-fed are less likely to develop diabetes and ear infections. However, if a woman has HIV, the virus that causes AIDS, she should not breast-feed, since the HIV virus will be in the breast milk.

Some relatives or friends give a mother-to-be a baby shower to help her gather the items her baby will need. The parents may register or select items at a store of their choice. Another option for helping to lower the costs of an infant is to shop at secondhand stores or consignment shops that carry baby and infant items. They carry almost all of a baby's needs at a much lower price.

Another thing to consider is child care. Some parents need to work outside the home or attend school after having a baby. Placing a baby in day care can be expensive and can be a big financial shock to new parents. Some parents choose to have a baby-sitter watch their child. Baby-sitters usually charge by the hour. Other parents choose to place their child in a day care center. At these centers, one or more persons watch several children. Some places care for fewer than 10 children, while others are responsible for several hundred. Full-time day care can cost $100 or more a week. This can total more than $5,000 a year.

Q & A

Question: What are my rights for parental leave from work?

Answer: The U.S. Congress passed the Family and Medical Leave Act in 1993. If you or your husband has spent at least one year working for a company, the law allows each of you to take up to 12 weeks of unpaid leave in any 12-month period for the birth of your baby. Leave may be taken from time to time or all at once. However, the act applies only to companies that employ 50 or more people within a 75-mile radius. States also have laws about parental leave, and they differ. To find out if your workplace is covered, check with your state labor office or consult your company's human resources department.

TEEN MOTHERS AND WELFARE

According to the National Campaign to Prevent Teen and Unplanned Pregnancy, teen mothers on welfare accounted for at least $2.3 billion in costs in 2006. Welfare is a government-organized effort to provide financial assistance to needy families. Within five years of having their first baby, almost one-half of all teenage mothers and 75 percent of unmarried teen mothers are on welfare. Taking care of a child is expensive, and most teens cannot do it on their own without support from their families or welfare.

New moms are under a huge amount of financial stress, which comes as no surprise as American families struggle to cover the cost of health care, housing, and higher education.

TEENS SPEAK

Unexpected Costs

I'm 19 years old, I have two kids and they'll be four this month. They are twins; a boy and a girl named Damien and Zoe. I got pregnant when I was just a freshman in high school. It was rough telling my mom and it was hard to fit behind my desk at school when I put on 80 pounds. Most of all, I didn't know how much it would cost to deliver my babies. Just having my kids, and going to the hospital cost $4,000, and the average cost of having a baby is nearly $2,500 a month.

AFFORDING A BABY

There are many financial costs of being pregnant, delivering a baby, and raising a baby. There is much to consider and plan for financially, including prenatal care, delivery care, and infant care. Being financially stable for this grand responsibility is important.

See also: Relationships and Responsibilities

FURTHER READING

American College of Obstetricians and Gynecologists (ACOG). *Planning Your Pregnancy and Birth*. 3rd ed. Washington, D.C.: ACOG 2002.

Boston Women's Health Book Collective and Judy Norsigian. *Our Bodies, Ourselves: Pregnancy and Birth*. New York: Touchstone, 2008.

Brott, Armin A., and Jennifer Ash. *The Expectant Father*. 2nd ed. New York: Abbeville Press, 2001.

■ PREGNANCY AND TEENAGERS

Pregnancy is the period of time in which a baby develops in the **uterus** (the female reproductive organ in which a fertilized egg is implanted and the fetus develops). In the United States about one million teenagers get pregnant each year, according to the Centers for Disease Control and Prevention (CDC) and the National Campaign to Prevent Teen and Unplanned Pregnancy.

According to the National Campaign, the U.S. teen pregnancy rate for teens aged 15–19 decreased 38 percent between 1990 and 2004. After reaching 117 pregnancies per 1,000 females aged 15–19 in 1990, the pregnancy rate has decreased to 72 pregnancies per 1,000 females aged 15–19 in 2004.

TOWARD A HEALTHY PREGNANCY

Teens who become pregnant experience a wide range of emotions. Many did not plan to have a baby. Some are worried about how the news will affect their relationship with the baby's father, their own parents, and their friends. Whether a pregnant woman feels confused, worried, scared, or excited, her life is about to change. The choices she makes over the next few months will greatly affect her own future and the future of her baby.

Prenatal care

Prenatal care is the medical care a woman and her baby need during pregnancy. The sooner a woman receives medical care, the better the chances that she and her baby will be healthy. Those who cannot afford a doctor or clinic should consult a social service organization. School guidance counselors, parents, a family doctor, or other trusted adults can help in locating community resources.

During the first visit, the doctor asks lots of questions to help him or her estimate how far along the woman is in the pregnancy and a possible due date. The doctor will also examine the expectant mother and perform a variety of exams and tests. If the doctor is aware of sexually transmitted diseases and other medical problems early in the pregnancy, he or she can help the expectant mother protect the baby as it develops.

The doctor should explain the physical and emotional changes a woman can expect during pregnancy. He or she can also teach an expectant mother how to recognize signs of a possible complication. This is especially important, because teens are more at risk for certain complications such as high blood pressure, miscarriage, and premature labor.

The doctor will also start the expectant mother on prenatal vitamins that contain folic acid, calcium, and iron. Many of these vitamins help protect against birth defects.

That first visit is just the beginning. The doctor will usually want to see an expectant mother once a month for the first 28 weeks of pregnancy, then every two to three weeks until 36 weeks, then once a week until the baby is born. If the expectant mother has a medical condition that may affect the baby, the doctor may wish to see her more often.

One important part of prenatal care is attending classes where expectant mothers can learn about having a healthy pregnancy and delivery as well as the basics of caring for a new baby. These classes may be offered at local hospitals, clinics, schools, or colleges.

Changes to expect during pregnancy

Pregnancy causes many physical changes in the body. The following are some of the most common changes:

- An increase in breast size
- Changes in the skin, including acne and brownish or yellowish patches on the face and the lower abdomen as a result of pregnancy hormones

- Mood swings, including depression during pregnancy and after delivery
- Discomfort, including nausea and vomiting, leg swelling, hemorrhoids, heartburn and constipation, backache, fatigue, and loss of sleep

During pregnancy, a woman should check with her doctor before taking any medication, including over-the-counter medications, herbal remedies, and vitamins. Smoking, drinking, and taking drugs are never a good idea, but they are particularly dangerous during pregnancy. They put not only the expectant mother but also her baby at risk of serious physical and mental problems. An expectant mother should ask her doctor for help if she is trying to quit smoking, drinking, or doing drugs.

Expectant mothers should also avoid dieting during pregnancy. Both they and their babies need certain nutrients to grow properly. Good nutrition and exercise are essential.

ISSUES INVOLVING PREGNANCY

Teens who become parents often face a variety of problems, including difficulties in completing their education and limited employment opportunities. They also face a variety of health problems associated with early childbearing.

In 2008, the March of Dimes reported that only 40 percent of teen mothers finished high school. About 64 percent graduate or receive a GED within two years of the date on which they would have graduated with their class, compared to 75 percent of teenage women who did not give birth. By age 30, only 1.5 percent of teen mothers had earned a college degree. Included in those statistics are teens who left high school for a reason other than pregnancy but later became pregnant.

All of the research indicates that women who complete high school are more likely to have good jobs and enjoy more success in their lives. Most school counselors can help pregnant teens find information about classes and programs in their community that provide support for teen parents. Some high schools have child-care centers on campus.

According to Planned Parenthood, only 63 percent of teens who give birth before age 18 and 74 percent of teens who give birth between ages 18 and 19 either graduate from high school or receive their GED—as compared to approximately 85 percent of women who

Teen Birth Rates in 2005

Country	Rate (Per 1,000 women ages 15–19)
Netherlands	4.6
Japan	5.6
France	7.8
Germany	11.0
Canada	14.5
Australia	16.1
United States	40.4

Source: Planned Parenthood.

delay childbirth until their early twenties. One reason that many teen mothers drop out of school is the need to work in order to support their child. Most cannot manage parenthood, school, and a job without the support of family and friends. Babies require constant care. Some teens turn to various government programs to help them make it through their baby's first years. **Welfare** is a term used to describe government assistance to needy families. Welfare recipients include those who are unable to work as well as those who do have jobs but do not earn enough money to support themselves or their families.

Medicaid is a federal and state health insurance program designed to provide access to health services for persons below a certain income level. (Income levels for eligibility vary with the cost of living in a particular community.) Teens may be eligible for Medicaid if they or their families cannot afford the costs associated with having a baby. Medicaid covers about 80 percent of all teen births in the United States according to the National Campaign to Prevent Teen Pregnancy in 2003.

Health problems
Young teens (those who are under the age of 15) and their babies may face serious health problems as a result of a pregnancy. According to Advocates for Youth, those problems include the following:

- Adolescent females seem to be more susceptible to sexually transmitted diseases (STDs) than older women. Teen girls have fewer antibodies to STDs and may therefore have a higher risk of cervical infections.

- The death rate in childbirth for teens under the age of 15 is two and a half times greater than for mothers who are between the ages of 20 and 24.

- Babies born to teens younger than 15 are more than twice as likely to be low-birth-weight babies—babies under 5.5 pounds at birth—and three times more likely to die in the first 28 days of life than babies born to older mothers.

In 2003, the Guttmacher Institute, a group that researches issues related to health and public education, found that approximately 7 percent of teen mothers did not receive adequate prenatal care. As a result, their babies experienced more childhood health problems than those born to older women. The link between early childbearing and the health of the infant is not due to the age of the mother but to the many risk factors associated with her youth, such as inadequate nutrition. The younger a woman is when she becomes pregnant, the less likely she is to seek prenatal care during her first trimester.

To compound the problem, many young teens are not fully developed before getting pregnant. Therefore, they may not be able to nourish their babies without taking away nutrients needed for their own growing bodies. The nutrients an expectant mother consumes go to the developing baby, thereby depleting nutrients needed for her own growth. Pregnant teens are also more at risk for a miscarriage, toxemia (blood poisoning), and hemorrhaging (excessive bleeding).

In 2008, the March of Dimes reported that studies indicate that 78 percent of children born to an unmarried teenage high-school dropout live in poverty and are 50 percent more likely to repeat a grade in school. Daughters of teen mothers themselves are 22 percent more likely to become teen mothers. In addition, children of teen parents are also twice as likely to be the victim of abuse and neglect.

TEENS SPEAK

I Have a Baby, and
I Can't Give Him All He Needs

I'm 16 and have a three-month-old boy. At first I thought I could handle it and give my son all he needed. Now I realize I can't. I have no job because I have to take care of him after school.

My mom watches him during the day so I can finish school. I feel like I have to rely on her to buy him everything. There are things I want to get for him that I can't afford.

I get so frustrated when he cries and screams. I don't know what to do to make him stop. Sometimes I just want to shake him. I know I can't, because I could really hurt him. He doesn't know what he is doing and can't tell me what's wrong, so I know it's not his fault. I just wish I had more patience.

There are nights when I get no sleep at all. I'm up all night and then I have to go to school the next morning. My friends think he is so cute. He is, but they have no idea how hard it really is. If I had known, I never would have had unprotected sex. I'm lucky in that I get help from my family. I can't imagine doing this all on my own.

CULTURAL ISSUES WITH
TEENAGE PREGNANCY

According to the Guttmacher Institute in a 2006 report, each year almost 750,000 women aged 15–19 become pregnant. Overall, 75 pregnancies occur every year per 1,000 women aged 15–19; this rate has declined 36 percent since its peak in 1990.

According to Advocates for Youth and the Guttmacher Institute, the United States has the highest teen pregnancy and teen birth rate among developed countries. The Guttmacher Institute conducted a study in 2006 that compared teens in the United States with such nations as Sweden, Germany, and France. Researchers found that rates of teen sexual activity are about the same in all four nations.

However, teens in Sweden, Germany, and France were more likely to use birth control, had greater access to contraceptives, experienced less peer pressure to have sex, and received more sexuality education than American teens.

For teens, it may be more difficult to be parents and provide quality parenting. Many teens may not be emotionally and physically ready to be parents. Others don't have the skills or time to dedicate to parenting with school to finish.

Q & A

Question: Will my boyfriend stay with me if we have a baby?

Answer: The National Campaign to Prevent Teen and Unplanned Pregnancy states that only about 20 percent of teen fathers actually stay with the mother and help to raise the baby. Your boyfriend may have good intentions at first and say he will stay with you, but things can change. It is easier for the male to leave since he doesn't have to carry and deliver the baby. He is not tied to the baby like the mother is.

Why do teens get pregnant?

Teens get pregnant for a variety of reasons, including peer pressure to have sex, lack of knowledge or resources to prevent pregnancy, or simply wanting a baby. Some teens may want to remain abstinent but not know how to tell their partner no. The teen pregnancy rate is down, due to more consistent contraceptive use; also due to higher proportions of teens choosing to delay sexual activity. According to the Youth Risk Behavior Surveillance System in 2007, approximately 60 percent of teens reported using a condom during their last intercourse experience. Of the nearly one-half that did not use contraceptives, some wanted to get pregnant. They may believe that a baby will bring them the love they may not be getting at home or help them to keep a boyfriend.

Male cultural issues

In American society, many teen males feel pressure to be sexually active. Males may not know how to resist that pressure. Of those who decide to become sexually active, many are not prepared to use a contraceptive or they may expect their partner to assume responsibility for birth control. By not using a condom, males put themselves and their partners at risk of an unwanted pregnancy or STD.

Female cultural issues

Females in American society are still faced with the double standard. They are not expected to carry condoms and may appear "bad" if they seem prepared for sex.

Females are also expected to be nurturing and caring. Just because they may make good mothers in the future doesn't mean they are ready as teens. Both females and males make better parents when they have had the opportunity to learn about themselves and others. As people age, the experiences they have help them to mature and learn patience. It takes time and experience to become a good mother or father and truly understand what children need.

WHY WAITING IS IMPORTANT

Many teenagers in the United States are becoming parents before they complete their education or enjoy an active social life. The quality of parenting is negatively affected when someone raises a child without learning life skills themselves. The health and the quality of life of the baby may be affected. Parenting is a full-time job that requires patience, maturing, financial stability, and time.

See also: Conception, Pregnancy, and Childbirth; Prenatal Care

FURTHER READING

Steinberg, Laurence D. *Adolescence.* 6th ed. Boston: McGraw-Hill, 2002.

■ PRENATAL CARE

The healthcare, education, and counseling that a woman receives before and during pregnancy. According to the National Institutes of Health, getting early and regular prenatal care is important for both the mother and the developing baby. Prenatal care helps a woman handle different aspects of pregnancy. Health experts recommend that women initiate prenatal care in the first three months of pregnancy. Early prenatal care can be beneficial through early identification of risk factors; treatment of conditions such as **diabetes** and high blood pressure; and referrals to services such as nutrition and smoking cessation programs.

Prenatal care helps improve maternal health and survival and may contribute to improved infant survival by linking women with high-risk pregnancies to better pre- and postnatal care. Mothers who obtain adequate prenatal care are more likely to obtain preventive care for their infants, increasing the chances for good health throughout childhood. Prenatal care also includes the discussion of many other issues, such as nutrition and physical activity, what to expect during the birth process, and basic skills for caring for an infant.

According to the Centers for Disease Control and Prevention, almost 4 million U.S. women give birth every year. Nearly one third of them will have some kind of pregnancy-related complication. The risk for complications during pregnancy is higher in women who do not receive adequate prenatal care. This can lead to potentially serious consequences for both the mother and her baby. The sooner in the pregnancy that a woman begins to receive prenatal care, the better the chances of ensuring the health of the expectant mother and of the baby. More women are seeking early care: According to the Child Trends DataBank, the percentage of births to women receiving late or no prenatal care declined from 6.1 percent in 1990 to 3.6 percent by 2004.

CARE BEFORE CONCEPTION

Ideally, prenatal care should start before the woman gets pregnant. Women who are planning a pregnancy should see their health care provider for a complete checkup. He or she can do routine testing to make sure the woman is in good health and that she doesn't have any illnesses or other conditions that could affect the pregnancy.

The goal of prenatal care is to monitor the progress of a pregnancy and to identify potential problems before they become serious for either the mother or the baby. A woman with a preexisting condition such as diabetes, asthma, high blood pressure, or heart problems should discuss these conditions with a physician to find out how the pregnancy could be affected.

Some women enroll in childbirth education classes that are designed to help the women draft a birth plan—a written outline of what they would like to have happen during labor and delivery. This plan may include the setting each woman wants to give birth in, the people the woman would want to have with her, and the pain medications the woman would want, if any.

Healthy behaviors

For the baby's and the mother's sake, it is important to follow the basics: don't smoke, drink alcohol, or take drugs. Expectant mothers should get plenty of rest and eat a healthy diet. Receiving care before conception allows the woman to also talk to the doctor about healthy behaviors. Doctors generally recommend that women add about 300 calories to their daily intake to provide nourishment for the developing fetus. Although protein should supply most of these calories, the diet needs to be well balanced, including fresh fruits, grains, and vegetables. If you or your partner has a family history of a significant genetic disorder and you suspect either of you may be a carrier, then genetic testing may be advisable.

Pregnant women should also avoid eating shark, swordfish, king mackerel, or tilefish. Although fish and shellfish can be an extremely healthy part of a woman's pregnancy diet (they contain beneficial omega-3 fatty acids and are high in protein and low in saturated fat), these types of fish may contain high levels of mercury, which can cause damage to the developing brain of a fetus.

VITAMINS

Prenatal supplements consist of a variety of vitamins and minerals. During pregnancy, a woman's daily intake requirements for certain nutrients, such as folic acid (folate), calcium, and iron, will increase. Vitamins and minerals such as iron, calcium, and folic acid are vital for proper fetal growth, development, and healthy adult living. Folic acid is very important for women who are planning to become pregnant because neural tube defects happen in the first 28 days of pregnancy, often before a woman even knows she's pregnant.

Over-the-counter medications are generally considered off-limits because of their potential effects on the fetus. Most doctors will recommend that a pregnant woman not take any over-the-counter medications at all, but they might offer a list of those they think are safe to take.

FIRST VISIT AND ROUTINE VISITS

During the first prenatal care visit, the provider will ask a lot of questions and do some tests. All women need prenatal care. Women who see a healthcare provider regularly during pregnancy have healthier babies, are less likely to deliver prematurely, and are less likely to have other serious problems related to pregnancy. A typical prenatal care schedule for a low-risk woman with a normally progressing

DID YOU KNOW?

How a Baby Grows

The First Trimester: 0–13 Weeks

- The placenta develops
- The major organs and nervous system form
- The heart starts beating
- The lungs begin to develop
- Bones appear
- The head, face, eyes, ears, arms, fingers, legs, and toes form
- Hair starts to grow
- Buds for 20 temporary teeth develop

The Second Trimester: 14–28 Weeks

- The organs develop further and begin to function
- Eyebrows, eyelashes, and fingernails form
- The skin is wrinkled and covered with a waxy coating
- The genitals develop
- Fine hair covers the body
- The fetus moves, kicks, sleeps, and wakes
- The fetus can swallow, hear, pass urine, and suck its thumb

The Third Trimester: 29–40 Weeks

- The fetus kicks and stretches
- Fine body hair disappears
- The fetus gains most of its weight—about half a pound each week until birth
- Bones harden, but the skull remains soft and flexible for delivery

Adapted with permission from American College of Obstetricians and Gynecologists.

pregnancy encourages one visit per month for the first 28 weeks, followed by two visits per month up to 36 weeks.

The doctor or nurse will do the following: ask about health history, including diseases, operations, or prior pregnancies; ask about family health history; do a complete physical exam; do a pelvic exam; order tests of blood and urine samples; check blood pressure, urine, height, and weight; figure out the expected due date; and answer questions.

At the first visit, the woman should ask questions and discuss any issues related to the pregnancy. Later prenatal visits will probably be shorter. The doctor will check on the woman's health and make sure the baby is growing as expected. Most prenatal visits will include checking the baby's heart rate, checking the woman's blood pressure, checking the woman's urine for signs of diabetes, and measuring the woman's weight gain during pregnancy.

After 36 weeks, women are strongly encouraged to continue visits once per week until birth. A woman with a chronic medical condition or a "high-risk" pregnancy may have to see her health care provider more often.

An **ultrasound** (also called a sonogram, sonograph, echogram, or ultrasonogram) is usually performed at 18 to 20 weeks to look at the baby's anatomy. It can be done sooner or later and sometimes more than once. It poses no risk to the mother and the baby. The ultrasound examination is done to make sure the pregnancy is progressing normally and to verify the expected date of delivery. A technician will coat the woman's abdomen with a gel and then run a wandlike instrument over it. High-frequency sound waves "echo" off the baby's body and create a picture of the fetus on a computer screen.

Fact Or Fiction?

Teenage mothers are less likely to get prenatal care.

The Facts: According to the Centers for Disease Control and Prevention, when teens give birth, their future prospects and those of their children decline. Teen mothers are less likely to complete high school and more likely to live in poverty than other teens. Pregnant teens aged 15–19 years are less likely to receive prenatal care and gain appropriate weight and more likely to smoke than pregnant women aged 20 years or older.

About one-third of girls in the United States get pregnant before age 20. In 2006, a total of 435,427 infants were born to mothers aged 15–19 years. These factors are also associated with poor birth outcomes.

See also: Birth Defect and Risk-Taking Behaviors; Pregnancy and Teenagers

FURTHER READING
American College of Obstetricians and Gynecologists. "You and Your Baby: Prenatal Care, Labor and Delivery, and Postpartum Care." ACOG Education Pamphlet AB005, January 2007. Available online. URL: http://www.acog.org/publications/patient_education/ab005. cfm. Accessed January 12, 2009.
American Pregnancy Association. Available online. URL: http://www. americanpregnancy.org/index.htm. Accessed January 12, 2009.

■ RAPE
See: Violence, Sexual

■ RELATIONSHIPS AND RESPONSIBILITIES
Connections of friendship or kinship between individuals. In any relationship, whether or not it's sexual, each person has responsibilities to the other. In a sexual relationship, each partner is responsible for communicating clearly, showing respect for one's partner, and sharing the responsibility of contraception.

HEALTHY AND UNHEALTHY RELATIONSHIPS
In healthy relationships, people are supportive, kind, and show friendship to one another. Neither person feels scared of or uncomfortable with the other. They complement each other and make each other feel happy and safe.

Fights, arguments, and even physical aggression often characterize unhealthy relationships. One partner may be fearful of the other. He or she may also be afraid of upsetting the other person. Unhealthy relationships may be controlling and can sometimes be dangerous. Some teens know they are in an unhealthy relationship, but stay in it because they are afraid to get out or do not know how to get out.

MAKING RESPONSIBLE DECISIONS

Partners in a sexual relationship make joint decisions. Those decisions may include choosing whether to abstain from sex, selecting a birth control method that satisfies both partners, and finding a way to protect one another from **sexually transmitted diseases** (STDs), diseases that are spread through sexual contact. In making such decisions, each person should consider his or her own values regarding sex and engage only in activities he or she is comfortable with. If either partner has questions about sex, he or she should talk with parents, friends, or other people they trust. Ultimately, however, the decision is personal—what seems right for one teen may not be right for another.

Becoming a good decision maker requires practice in making choices and communicating one's needs to others. Being strong enough to stand up for one's beliefs is crucial. By standing up for themselves, individuals learn how to protect themselves and to question anything that makes them uncomfortable. Everyone should learn to trust his or her instincts. Some people may try to convince a person to change a decision. However, one usually knows what is the best decision for oneself.

Making a difficult decision

All decisions have consequences, some good and some bad. When faced with a decision, the following technique can be useful in sorting out ones thoughts. Think of the acronym "SOCS," which stands for situation, options, consequences, and solution. Describe the difficult situation on a sheet of paper. Next list the options. Then write the consequences for each option. Writing this information may help you find a solution that works for you. Most situations have a variety of possible ones.

Many factors impact a person's decision making. A decision that seemed right at one point in a person's life may not seem right a few years later. Attitudes change and feelings alter as one grows older and becomes more mature. Change is normal. A poor decision in the past does not have to limit choices today or tomorrow. Although the past can't be changed, the future can be altered.

Self-esteem

Self-esteem is a personal feeling of self worth. People with high self-esteem trust themselves and have faith in their decisions. They tend to be proud of themselves and have confidence in their abilities. They are usually good at communicating their needs to others and are able to stand up for themselves.

People with low self-esteem may question their capabilities and have difficulty making decisions. They may have it hard to state their needs and may allow others to take advantage of them by not standing up for themselves.

Q & A

Question: What if your partner wants sex, but you're not sure you're ready?

Answer: Sex is a big decision. You and your partner may want different things from a relationship. If you are not ready for sex, tell your partner. You can explain that you care about him or her and still say "no" or "not yet" to sex. A partner who respects you and truly cares about you will wait.

Alcohol and drugs in decision making

Alcohol and drugs impact judgment skills. Alcohol consumption, for example, causes a number of marked changes in behavior. Even low doses significantly impair the judgment and coordination needed to drive a car safely. Low to moderate doses of alcohol may result in a variety of aggressive acts, including partner and child abuse. Moderate to high doses of alcohol may damage a person's ability to learn and remember information.

When people are under the influence of drugs or alcohol, they may not be aware of the consequences of their actions. Faulty judgment may lead to a loss of inhibition, which in turn may, in some people, result in an increase in violent behaviors. The potential physical effects of drugs and alcohol on the body also include poor motor coordination, irritability, and blurred vision.

When a person is drunk, saying "no" to unwanted sexual behavior may be more difficult. He or she may not be thinking clearly and may fail to consider the risk of contracting an STD or becoming pregnant.

Some individuals think they are invincible and act like they will live forever. Others become violent. The combination of a loss of judgment, impaired vision, impaired coordination, and irritability, can be deadly. U.S. government statistics indicate that at least one-half of all incidences of domestic violence, assault, and homicide are associated with the consumption of alcohol and other drugs.

COMMUNICATE TO MAKE DECISIONS

Responsible decision makers communicate with their partner. Communication skills can help people in a relationship describe their feelings and their needs. Talking about thoughts, emotions, and feelings can be difficult. Many people learn to communicate as they go. Some helpful hints for improving communication include the four L's of communication: listening, looking, leveling, and loving.

- Listening. Many people think they are listening when they really are not. A person may hear what his or her partner is saying but fail to understand what he or she means. Good listeners pay attention. They try to put themselves in the other person's shoes by attempting to understand his or her thoughts and feelings. One way to do so is by restating or rephrasing what the speaker has said or by relating what they hear to what they already know. They also avoid cutting speakers off before they finish what they have to say.

- Looking. Good listeners pay attention to nonverbal messages—the tone of the speaker's voice, their facial expressions, posture, gestures, and even energy level.

- Leveling. Being honest with a partner means telling the truth. Lying to make oneself or one's partner feel better for the moment is not worth the effort. Being honest does not mean being rude. To be polite, always take responsibility for your feelings. Instead of saying "You always . . . " try saying "I feel . . . " or "I think . . . " Such statements make the other person feel less threatened and more willing to listen.

- Loving. Sometimes people hold back their true feelings because they think their partner does not care. Expressing love is an important part of communication and also helps with healing.

Sharing the responsibility for contraception

If a couple decides to have sex, one major decision they should make is whether they want to have a child at the present time. If not, they may want to decide on a method of **contraception,** or birth control. Being prepared shows that a couple is responsible and has thought about the consequences.

Protection from a sexually transmitted disease or an unwanted pregnancy is the responsibility of both partners in a relationship. It should not be a decision that only one person makes. Although bringing up the topic may not be easy, it should be discussed ahead of time. Waiting until the couple is about to have sex is too late. Talking with a partner about protection and sex builds trust. Couples who have not reached that level of trust may not be ready for sex.

TEENS SPEAK

We Didn't Use Protection

About a year ago my girlfriend and I had a bad experience. We had sex for the first time and didn't use protection. We hadn't ever talked about it. I didn't know how to bring it up. I knew we would eventually have sex; I just thought we'd talk about it ahead of time. I also assumed I'd be more prepared. Not so.

I didn't have a condom with me the night we had sex. When things got hot, I asked her if she was on the pill. She said "no" but didn't stop me. She told me to "just pull out." I thought I'd have more control than I did that night. I wasn't able to withdraw in time. I was so embarrassed and scared. For a few days that seemed like eternity, I was scared to death that she was pregnant.

We talked about what we would do if she were pregnant. We also talked about what contraceptive to use in the future. Luckily she got her period a few days later. It took being scared out of our minds to talk about it. We were lucky. It could have been too late.

GETTING ACCURATE INFORMATION

People need accurate information to make responsible decisions. Not everything one reads, sees on television, hears on the radio, or hears from other people is correct. Many sexuality-related myths exist. Examples include "You can't get pregnant the first time" and "You can't get pregnant if a girl is having her period." Both of these myths, and many others, come from people who do not know the facts. People need to be skeptical and ask tough questions rather than believe everything they hear.

For reliable sources of information about sexuality, many people turn to the Centers for Disease Control and Prevention (CDC), Planned Parenthood, and the National Campaign to Prevent Pregnancy. These groups have informative publications and Web sites. In addition, most public libraries contain books on sexuality written by experts in the field.

Reliable sources on the Internet

Anyone can post information on the Internet, so one should pay attention to the sources of that information. Who sponsors the site? Who wrote the article? What proof does the author use to support his or her opinions? A few of the sexuality-related sites where one can find reliable and accurate information include:

- www.goaskalice.com. Sponsored by the University of South Carolina, this is a place where teens can ask questions and get real answers.

- www.plannedparenthood.org. This site contains information on sexuality from family planning to emergency contraception. It keeps up with the latest sexuality information and facts.

- www.cdc.gov. The Centers for Disease Control and Prevention (CDC) offers a variety of "fact sheets" on popular topics and information on medical conditions.

- www.siecus.org. The Sexuality Information and Education Council of the United States provides reliable information on sex education and sexuality.

- www.thenationalcampaign.org. The National Campaign to Prevent Teen and Unplanned Pregnancy contains accurate, up-to-date information on teen pregnancy and relationships.

Each of these Web sites is linked to other reliable sites. When viewing other sites, check to see who sponsors the Web site or authors the articles. The author should be a professional, such as a physician. The sponsoring site should be a professional organization, such as the American School Health Association, or a department of a state or the federal government, such as the Department of Health and Human Services.

MAKING GOOD DECISIONS IN RELATIONSHIPS
People in relationships have responsibilities to themselves and their partners. Good decision making is critical to establishing, maintaining, and deepening relationships. Teens are faced with many difficult situations and have many questions regarding sex and relationships. By trusting their instincts, communicating their needs effectively to their partners, and relying on accurate and reliable information, teens will be able to make the best decision possible.

See also: Dating; Pregnancy, Prevention of; Sex and the Law

FURTHER READING
Christensen, Andrew, and Neil Jacobson. *Reconcilable Differences.* New York: Guilford Press, 2000.
Fletcher, Garth. *The New Science of Intimate Relationships.* Oxford: Blackwell, 2002.
Miller, Rowland, and Daniel Perlman. *Intimate Relationships.* 5th ed. Columbus, Ohio: McGraw-Hill, 2009.

■ REPRODUCTION
See: Conception, Pregnancy, and Childbirth

■ SEX AND THE LAW
Laws related to sexuality and sexual behaviors exist in every state but differ slightly. Many of these laws focus on the most basic decisions

Americans make about their lives—marriage and divorce, childbearing, and sexual conduct.

SEXUAL ACTIVITY

Every state bans some sexual activities and permits others. These laws reflect the values and beliefs of the state and its people.

Sodomy laws

Until 1969, every state in the United States had **sodomy laws** (laws that make oral and anal sex between consenting adults illegal). Some banned sodomy only between partners of the same sex. Others banned sodomy for both heterosexual and homosexual couples. Over the years, little by little, those laws have been repealed or blocked by state courts in 37 states.

In November 2003, the U.S. Supreme Court overturned Texas's sodomy law and in doing so declared similar laws in 12 other states unconstitutional. In writing the decision of the majority, Justice Anthony Kennedy noted, "The petitioners are entitled to respect for their private lives. The state cannot demean their existence or control their destiny by making their private sexual conduct a crime."

A matter of consent

In overturning these laws, the courts argued that private sexual conduct should not be a crime unless one of the participants objects. Most states use the term **sexual assault** to describe all forced sexual contact, including **rape.** Rape is forced sexual penetration. Some states substitute the term *aggravated sexual assault* for "rape," and many states include homosexual rape, incest (sexual intercourse between persons too closely related to marry, as between a parent and a child), and other sex offenses in a definition of rape.

In most states, the courts have ruled that people who are under the influence of alcohol or drugs cannot give their consent to sexual activity. Therefore, **drug-facilitated rape** is considered rape. Both parties must agree to have sex. Anyone who is drunk cannot legally give consent. Just because a person doesn't say no doesn't mean that he or she is saying yes. In some situations, like being under the influence of drugs or alcohol, an individual may not be physically able to say no, even though he or she does not want sex.

DID YOU KNOW?

Age of Consent by State

State	Age	State	Age
Alabama	16	Montana	16
Alaska	16	Nebraska	16
Arizona	18	Nevada	16
Arkansas	16	New Hampshire	16
California	18	New Jersey	16
Colorado	17	New Mexico	16
Connecticut	16	New York	17
Delaware	18	North Carolina	16
District of Columbia	16	North Dakota	18
Florida	18	Ohio	16
Georgia	16	Oklahoma	16
Hawaii	16	Oregon	18
Idaho	18	Pennsylvania	16
Illinois	17	Rhode Island	16
Indiana	16	South Carolina	16
Iowa	16	South Dakota	16
Kansas	16	Tennessee	18
Kentucky	16	Texas	17
Louisiana	17	Utah	18
Maine	16	Vermont	16
Maryland	16	Virginia	18
Massachusetts	16	Washington	16
Michigan	16	West Virginia	16
Mississippi	16	Wisconsin	18
Missouri	17	Wyoming	16
Minnesota	16		

Source: The Lewin Group, *Statutory Rape: A Guide to State Laws and Reporting Requirements,* 2004.

Sexual activity and the age of consent

People who are under the influence of drugs or alcohol cannot legally consent to sexual intercourse. Many state lawmakers believe that children also cannot legally consent to sex. Sex with a person who has not reached the age of consent is considered **statutory rape,** a crime in many states. In most, it is 18 years of age. Even if the underage person gives his or her consent, the older partner can be charged and prosecuted for statutory rape.

The average legal age of consent ranges from 16 to 18 years of age. In Ohio, the legal age of consent is 18. Therefore, if a 19-year-old male in Ohio has sex with his 17-year-old girlfriend, he can be charged with statutory rape. Although neither the young man nor his girlfriend may consider him a predator or rapist, the law says it is illegal for him or anyone else to have sex with her.

Some states are considering stronger enforcement of statutory rape laws and stronger punishments for people who commit statutory rape. According to the National Campaign to Prevent Teen Pregnancy, lawmakers in these states believe stronger enforcement will reduce the number of teen pregnancies, because adult men father over one-half of the babies born to teenagers. Other states are enforcing existing laws more strictly. Those states include California, Florida, Delaware, and Georgia.

Supporters of stronger enforcement suggest that if men know they risk prosecution, they may be less likely to have sex with a minor. Supporters also insist that enforcing existing laws may reduce adolescent pregnancy, since many adult males father several children by different teen mothers.

Other people believe that stronger statutory rape laws and more vigorous enforcement of those laws may have some negative outcomes. They may discourage sexually active and pregnant teens from seeking medical care if they fear their partner's age will lead to his arrest. They also feel that stronger laws may hurt healthy relationships between a teen and her adult male partner. Not all adult males who have babies with teen mothers are "predators" who seek to use young women for sex.

MARRIAGE

Every state in the nation has laws about who can marry and under what conditions. Although these laws vary slightly from state to state, they often include the following provisions:

- Marriage is a union of a husband and wife
- A minimum age (usually 18, though some states permit marriages at a younger age with the parents' consent)

- Not being too closely related to the intended spouse (All states prohibit a person from marrying a sibling, half-sibling, parent, grandparent, great-grandparent, child, grandchild, great-grandchild, aunt, uncle, niece, or nephew. Some states have additional prohibitions, including restrictions on marriages between cousins.)

- Having sufficient mental capacity—that is, both partners must understand what they are doing and what consequences their actions may have

- Being sober at the time of the marriage

- Not being married to anyone else

- Getting a blood test (only in Connecticut, Georgia, Indiana, Massachusetts, Mississippi, Montana, Oklahoma, and the District of Columbia)

- Obtaining a marriage license

Premarital blood tests, in the states that still require them, check both partners for sexually transmitted diseases (STDs) or rubella (measles). The tests may also disclose the presence of genetic disorders. No state tests for HIV or AIDS. If either partner tests positive for an STD, some states may refuse to issue the couple a marriage license. Other states may allow the couple to marry as long as both partners are aware that the disease is present.

Currently, most states recognize marriage only as the union of one man and one woman, though this policy is being contested in many states. In 2004, as the result of a successful court battle for the right to marry, same-sex couples in Massachusetts won the right to legally wed. Connecticut's supreme court legalized same-sex marriage in October 2008. In May 2008, the California Supreme Court overturned a state ban on same-sex marriages. However, in November 2008, California voters passed a ballot measure banning same-sex marriage. Similar actions have taken place in a few communities in New Mexico and New York.

On April 3, 2009, Iowa became the third state to allow same-sex marriage. On April 7, 2009, Vermont became the fourth state to allow same-sex marriage; it is the first state to allow same-sex marriage by legislature action. On April 29, 2009, New Hampshire passed same-sex marriage legislation, which is now awaiting the governor's signature or veto. On May 6, Maine followed to become the fifth state to allow same-sex marriage.

The push to allow civil unions and/or same-sex marriages has troubled some Americans who view marriage as the union of a man and a woman. They have persuaded a number of states to enact laws in defense of marriage.

Congress has also taken a stand on same-sex marriage. In 1996, it passed the Defense of Marriage Act. The law not only allows the

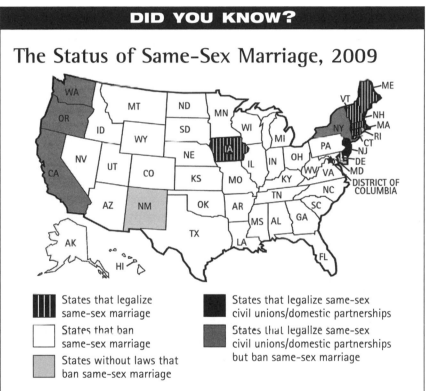

DID YOU KNOW?

The Status of Same-Sex Marriage, 2009

	States that legalize same-sex marriage
	States that ban same-sex marriage
	States without laws that ban same-sex marriage
	States that legalize same-sex civil unions/domestic partnerships
	States that legalize same-sex civil unions/domestic partnerships but ban same-sex marriage

Maine, New Hampshire, Vermont, Massachusetts, Connecticut, and Iowa legalize same-sex marriages. New Jersey allows civil unions. The District of Columbia, California, Oregon, New York, and Washington State recognize domestic partnerships. The 1996 Defense of Marriage Act effectively bars the federal government from recognizing same-sex unions, but marriages are certified by states, not the federal government.

Source: Human Rights Campaign, 2009.

federal government to refuse to recognize same-sex marriages but also gives states the right to refuse to recognize same-sex marriages licensed in other states. The law seems to contradict the U.S. Constitution, which requires that each state give "full faith and credit" to the laws of other states. For example, in the past, a couple who married in Massachusetts could be confident that their marriage would be legal in every other state. Now a married couple could find their marriage in question because of their sexual orientation. However, in May 2009, New York began recognizing marriages of same-sex couples who were married out of state.

DECISIONS ABOUT CONTRACEPTION AND ABORTION

Until 1973, **abortion** (the ending of a pregnancy) was illegal in most states within the United States. That year, the U.S. Supreme Court ruled in the case of *Roe v. Wade* that a woman has the right to decide whether to end or continue her pregnancy. A person's basic right to privacy includes a woman's decision to end her pregnancy. In a companion case, *Doe v. Bolton*, the Supreme Court ruled against a Georgia law that allowed abortions only if the pregnancy interfered with the health of the mother or in cases of rape and incest. The justices found that a woman has a constitutional right to abortion from six months to birth if her doctor "in his or her best clinical judgment," in light of the patient's age, "physical, emotional, psychological [and] familial" circumstances, finds it "necessary for her physical or mental health."

In the Court's view, the right to an abortion is not an unlimited right. The Court ruled that a woman has the right to choose until her **fetus** (the developing baby) is viable—which means that she can have an abortion until the pregnancy reaches a point where the fetus can survive outside the woman's body. At that time, a state may ban any abortion that is not necessary to preserve a woman's life or health.

As a result, abortions are legal in every state during the first trimester and illegal in every state during the third trimester. The only exceptions are if the mother's life is at risk or the fetus has severe abnormalities. Some states also deny abortions or place restrictions on them during the second trimester.

Q & A

Question: Can states pass laws that limit my right to use a contraceptive?

Answer: Until 1965, most states had laws that banned or limited access to contraceptives. In 1965, the U.S. Supreme Court ruled that the Constitution contains a "right to privacy" that protects the decision of married couples to use contraceptives. Therefore such bans or limitations are illegal. In 1972, the Court was asked whether individuals have the same right to acquire contraceptives that couples do. The justices ruled that they did. In 1977, the Court was asked whether people who are considered minors under the law have the right to purchase contraceptives and it ruled that they also have the right to do so.

The court's ruling has been controversial. Some groups have hailed the decision, noting that before abortions were legal, thousands were performed illegally, often under unsafe conditions. Opponents of abortion have worked over the years to limit the right to abortion, particularly for those who have not yet reached the age of consent.

Parental consent for abortions
Many states now require **parental consent** for an abortion. Parental consent is the approval of at least one parent prior to performing an abortion on a female under the age of 18. In other states, parental consent is not required. Other differences include the age of consent.

State laws regulate not only the age of consent but also the right of a teen to have an abortion. Approximately 30 states require notification of one or both parents before a young woman under 18 can have an abortion.

These laws assume that a pregnant teen has supportive, loving parents. Many teens do. Others have difficulty talking to their parents and may feel uncomfortable disclosing the pregnancy. Such leading medical groups as the American Medical Association and the American Academy of Pediatrics oppose laws requiring parental consent for abortion. Members believe that if the parents of a pregnant teen are unwilling to consent to an abortion, a teen may be forced to become a parent against her will.

DID YOU KNOW?

State Laws on Abortion

State	Parental involvement required	Mandatory delay following counseling required	Counseling required without mandatory delay	Insurance coverage restricted	State funding for Medicaid restricted
Alabama	Yes	Yes	No	No	Yes
Alaska	No	No	No	No	No
Arizona	Yes	No	No	No	No
Arkansas	Yes	No	No	No	Yes
California	No	No	Yes	No	No
Colorado	Yes	No	No	Yes	Yes
Connecticut	No	No	Yes	No	No
Delaware	Yes	No	No	No	Yes
District of Columbia	No	No	No	No	Yes
Florida	Yes	No	Yes	No	Yes
Georgia	Yes	Yes	No	No	Yes
Hawaii	No	No	No	No	No
Idaho	Yes	Yes	No	Yes	Yes
Illinois	No	No	No	Yes	No
Indiana	Yes	Yes	No	No	Yes
Iowa	Yes	No	No	No	Yes

Kansas	Yes	Yes	No	No	Yes
Kentucky	Yes	Yes	No	Yes	Yes
Louisiana	Yes	Yes	No	No	Yes
Maine	Yes	No	Yes	No	Yes
Maryland	Yes	No	No	No	No
Massachusetts	Yes	No	No	Yes	No
Michigan	Yes	Yes	No	No	Yes
Minnesota	Yes	No	Yes	No	No
Mississippi	Yes	Yes	No	Yes	Yes
Missouri	Yes	Yes	No	Yes	Yes
Montana	No	No	No	No	No
Nebraska	Yes	Yes	No	Yes	Yes
Nevada	No	No	Yes	No	Yes
New Hampshire	No	No	No	No	Yes
New Jersey	No	No	No	No	No
New Mexico	No	No	No	No	No
New York	No	No	No	No	No
North Carolina	Yes	No	No	No	Yes
North Dakota	Yes	Yes	No	Yes	Yes
Ohio	Yes	Yes	No	Yes	Yes
Oklahoma	Yes	Yes	No	Yes	Yes
Oregon	No	No	No	No	No
Pennsylvania	Yes	Yes	No	Yes	Yes

(continues)

DID YOU KNOW?

State Laws on Abortion (continued)

State	Parental involvement required	Mandatory delay following counseling required	Counseling required without mandatory delay	Insurance coverage restricted	State funding for Medicaid restricted
Rhode Island	Yes	No	Yes	Yes	Yes
South Carolina	Yes	Yes	No	Yes	Yes
South Dakota	Yes	Yes	No	No	No
Tennessee	Yes	No	No	No	Yes
Texas	Yes	Yes	No	No	Yes
Utah	Yes	Yes	No	No	Yes
Vermont	No	No	No	No	No
Virginia	Yes	Yes	No	Yes	Yes
Washington	No	No	No	No	No
West Virginia	Yes	Yes	No	No	No
Wisconsin	Yes	Yes	No	No	Yes
Wyoming	Yes	No	No	No	Yes

Source: The Guttmacher Institute, 2008.

In addition to parental consent, some states require counseling both with and without a mandatory delay. In these states, a woman seeking an abortion is required to get counseling related to her situation prior to receiving an abortion. In states that also require a mandatory delay, a woman is required to wait approximately 24 hours to contemplate her options before receiving an abortion. States also vary in the restrictions they place on insurance coverage for abortions. Some states restrict private insurance companies from covering abortions. Many states also restrict state funding for **Medicaid** to cover abortions. Medicaid is a taxpayer-funded, government-sponsored program that provides financial assistance for health needs.

KNOWING THE LAWS

State laws affect the most basic sexual choices a woman can make, including not only whether she can engage in sexual intercourse but also whether she can seek an abortion.

See also: Abortion; Sexual Predators; Violence, Sexual

FURTHER READING

Crooks, Robert, and Karla Baur. *Our Sexuality.* 7th ed. Pacific Grove, Calif.: Wadsworth Group, 2004.

■ SEXUAL AROUSAL

The arousal of sexual desires in preparation for sexual behavior. People all over the world have similar physical responses to sexual arousal. However, culture—the attitudes, values, and beliefs of a society, including its attitudes toward sexuality—also plays a role in what people find sexually arousing.

STANDARDS OF ATTRACTIVENESS

A people's culture shapes what they find attractive in others. Although physical appearance influences human sexual arousal in almost every culture, what is considered attractive varies greatly. For example, American men are among those who find bare female breasts arousing. In a number of other countries, including many African nations, people do not. Americans also consider a slender body attractive.

In other countries, men and women prefer partners who carry more weight.

THE EFFECT OF HORMONES

Hormones play a large role in sexual arousal. Hormones are chemical substances that regulate various functions in the body, including the reproductive organs and sexual motivation. Both males and females produce **testosterone** and **estrogen.**

Testosterone is a hormone associated with the development of not only **sperm,** or male sex cells, but also **secondary sex characteristics** and sex drive in both males and females. Secondary sex characteristics are the visible physical changes in males and females that occur as a result of increased hormones during puberty. Estrogen regulates reproductive functions and the development of secondary sex characteristics.

Men's bodies produce about 20–40 times more testosterone than women's. Testosterone has a greater impact on sexual desire, also known as libido, than on sexual functioning. Therefore, a man or woman with low testosterone levels may have little interest in sex but still able to become aroused and have an **orgasm.** An orgasm is pleasurable, rhythmic muscle contractions in the genital area resulting from sexual arousal.

Women's bodies produce more estrogen than men's bodies. In addition to maintaining the female reproductive structures, estrogen is responsible for breast development, the growth of hips, and patterns of hair growth. Estrogen also lowers **blood cholesterol levels.** A person's blood cholesterol level is the amount of **cholesterol,** a necessary waxy fatlike substance, in the blood. Higher estrogen levels in woman may be the reason women under 50 have a lower risk of heart disease than men their same age.

THE INFLUENCE OF THE BRAIN

The brain controls thoughts, emotions, memories, and fantasies. The way the brain responds to a stimulus, such as a picture, may differ from one person to the next. Seeing a sexually explicit image may sexually excite one person, while another may be turned off by the image or offended by it.

The **limbic system** is composed of several structures in the brain that influence the sexual behavior of humans and other animals. The **cerebral cortex** is the "thinking center" of the brain. It produces fantasies and is responsible for language, imagination, and reasoning. Together, the limbic system and the cerebral cortex play an important part in sexual arousal.

THE INFLUENCES OF THE SENSES

One's sense of touch, vision, smell, taste, and hearing also affect sexual arousal. Each person is unique and each has his or her own triggers of arousal.

An **erogenous zone** is a part of the body with many nerve endings and is therefore highly sensitive. These areas include the genitals, buttocks, breasts, thighs, stomach, neck, ears, hands, feet, and mouth. Not everyone likes to be touched in these places. Some may even find being touched in one or more of these places uncomfortable or irritating. Couples should discuss their likes and dislikes.

Sight can also be sexually arousing, although research suggests that women find visual stimuli less arousing than men do. In 1948 and again in 1953, Albert Kinsey, a noted expert in sexuality, completed the largest study of human sexual behavior ever conducted. He and his researchers found that men are more likely than women to be aroused by photos of attractive people.

Certain smells can also be arousing, depending on one's sexual history and cultural conditioning. For example, in the United States, some people are aroused by perfume or cologne. On the other hand, natural body odors may be more arousing for people from other cultures.

Sounds can also be arousing. Some people like to hear certain music, talk with their partners, or make noises during sexual activity. Others prefer silence.

Taste can also cause sexual arousal, although it may not be as powerful as the other senses. Certain products, like breath mints and flavored lubricants or lotions, may increase sexual arousal for some people.

Over the centuries, people in many cultures have insisted that a variety of **aphrodisiacs** increase sexual arousal. These are substances that stimulate desire or increase a person's capacity for sexual activities. Some people claim certain foods, such as oysters, bananas, celery, cucumbers, tomatoes, ginseng root, or potatoes are aphrodisiacs. The power of these foods seems to be a matter of belief and personal expectations rather than fact.

Some people believe alcohol increases sexual performance. In small amounts, alcohol may make one feel more at ease. That feeling may encourage him or her to approach a potential partner. In fact, alcohol is a depressant. It decreases sexual arousal and the ability to perform.

According to some people, illegal club drugs such as ecstasy heighten sexual arousal. Researchers have found no connection, although they have linked ecstasy to paranoia, liver damage, and heart attacks. They also note that the effects of club drugs are similar to those of alcohol. Both result in lowered sexual inhibitions, making users feel less shy and reserved. However, men generally cannot get erections while high on ecstasy.

THE IMPORTANCE OF FOREPLAY

Foreplay is any activity that contributes to sexual excitement. Foreplay may include kissing, touching, or oral sex. Foreplay does not always lead to sex. Some couples choose to simply enjoy foreplay without going further.

If a couple decides to have sex, foreplay helps both partners become physically ready. Although they may be prepared for sex emotionally, physical changes must occur in the body to make intercourse possible. With foreplay, the woman's vagina becomes lubricated and expands slightly. Without lubrication, sex would be uncomfortable and even painful. For men, foreplay causes an erection, the hardening of the penis necessary for intercourse.

Most couples enjoy foreplay as a healthy part of their physical relationship. It can help a couple discover what they mutually enjoy. Foreplay may also bring them closer and help them feel more comfortable with and trusting of each other.

VARIATIONS IN SEXUAL AROUSAL

Sexual arousal differs from one person to the next. Senses such as touch, smell, vision, and taste sexually arouse people differently. Hormones and foreplay affect arousal as well. Some people try to enhance arousal by using aphrodisiacs. When a person becomes sexually active, it is important to talk with his or her partner. Conversation helps couples discover each other's likes and dislikes while increasing comfort levels and trust.

See also: Biology and Sex; Media and Sex, The; Sexual Response

FURTHER READING
Ellison, Carol. *Women's Sexualities.* Oakland, Calif.: New Harbinger, 2000.

Heighway, Susan, and Susan Webster. *S.T.A.R.S.: A Social Skills Training Guide for Teaching Assertiveness, Relationship Skills, and Sexual Awareness*. Arlington, Tex.: Future Horizons, 2007.

McCarthy, Barry, and Emily McCarthy. *Male Sexual Awareness*. Berkeley, Calif.: Publishers Group West, 1998.

■ SEXUAL EXPRESSION

The attitudes and behaviors through which an individual reveals his or her sexual self. People express their sexuality in a variety of ways, based on personal preference, values, and comfort levels.

CELIBACY

Some people choose to not have sex. They prefer **celibacy**, or not engaging in sexual relations. People choose celibacy for a variety of reasons. Some believe that people should be married or in a committed relationship before having intercourse. Other individuals choose celibacy because it supports their religious or personal beliefs.

There are two types of celibacy: complete and partial. Those who practice **complete celibacy** do not **masturbate** or engage in any sexual activity with others. Masturbation is the stimulation of one's own genitals for sexual pleasure. **Partial celibacy** describes those who masturbate but do not engage in sexual behavior with another person.

A **virgin** is a person who has not yet had sex. Some teens choose to be virgins until they find the right person. Others hope to avoid the risks of unwanted pregnancy and sexually transmitted diseases (STDs).

Approximately one-half of all high school students are virgins. The Centers for Disease Control and Prevention (CDC) surveys students every year on six risk behaviors, one of which is sexual activity. In 2007, the Youth Risk Behavior Surveillance System (YRBSS) found that 67.2 percent of freshmen, 56.2 percent of sophomores, 44.5 percent of juniors, and 35.4 percent of seniors were virgins.

MASTURBATION

By the age of 20, almost all males and approximately three out of four females have masturbated, according to a 1997 study by the Sexuality Information and Education Council of the United States.

For some people, masturbation offers a release from sexual tension. Others masturbate to explore their own body and discover what they like. In the past, many people have felt guilty or embarrassed about masturbating. They were taught to believe it was wrong and even dangerous. Today experts maintain that masturbation is a healthy part of sexuality.

Fact Or Fiction?

Masturbation is harmful.

The Facts: Masturbation has no health risks. In the 1800s and early 1900s, many people believed masturbation caused blindness, stunted growth, led to memory loss, and damaged the body. Masturbation was considered evil. Today most people realize masturbation is not harmful and poses no health risks. Most physicians and other experts view masturbation as a healthy and positive way to express sexuality.

ORAL-GENITAL STIMULATION

Oral-genital stimulation, commonly referred to as oral sex, involves the use of the mouth and tongue to stimulate the sex organs. When

DID YOU KNOW?

Sexual Activity among U.S. High School Students

Grade	Percent who reported having had intercourse	Percent who reported having intercourse before age 13	Percent who reported having four or more partners
9	32.8	9.2	8.7
10	43.8	6.9	13.4
11	55.5	6.6	17.0
12	64.6	4.5	22.4
Total	47.8	7.1	14.9

Source: Centers for Disease Control and Prevention, 2007.

oral sex is performed on a woman, it is called **cunnilingus,** and when oral sex is performed on a man, it is called **fellatio.**

Some states have laws banning both oral sex and anal sex. These laws are known as **sodomy laws.** In 2003, the U.S. Supreme Court ruled that sodomy laws are unconstitutional, because individuals have a right to sexual privacy. The ruling affected the 13 states that still had sodomy laws, which applied primarily to gays and lesbians.

Some couples enjoy oral-genital stimulation, and others do not. Some individuals consider themselves to be virgins if they have had oral sex but not **intercourse,** vaginal or anal sex. However, oral sex is considered a form of sex. Although there is no risk of pregnancy, oral sex may put someone at risk of an STD.

Oral sex can be dangerous if performed on someone who has an STD. For example, people can get **gonorrhea,** a bacterial infection, or **herpes,** a viral infection causing painful, fluid-filled blisters on the mouth or in the throat. If a person has a sore on the mouth, such as a cold sore, he or she can pass it to a partner's genitals. There is also a possibility of transmitting **HIV,** the virus that causes AIDS, during oral sex if an open sore is present on a person's mouth.

The risk of STDs or HIV transmission during oral sex can be reduced if a man wears a condom while participating in oral sex. When performing oral sex on a woman, a **dental dam,** a piece of latex six inches square that is placed over a woman's entire genital area, can be used. Some people create a dental dam by cutting a condom lengthwise. By using protection during oral sex, one's mouth does not come in direct contact with a partner's genitals, greatly reducing the risk of STDs or HIV.

Q & A

Question: What happens if a woman swallows semen during oral sex?

Answer: Although she will not get pregnant or gain weight, she may be at risk of contracting an STD, including HIV. Some STDs are found in semen and vaginal fluids. A person is at risk for HIV if he or she has an open cut or sore in the mouth and gets semen or vaginal fluid in the mouth from a person who is HIV positive. Swallowing semen or vaginal fluid, according to the CDC, has not been proven to transmit HIV.

ANAL INTERCOURSE

Anal intercourse refers to a male putting his penis into the anus of a partner. Although it is more common among homosexual men, some heterosexual couples also have anal intercourse.

Anal intercourse is one of the riskiest sexual behaviors. Because the anus is composed of delicate tissue, it is more likely to tear than a vagina, increasing the risk of getting an STD. Therefore medical professionals recommend using a condom and additional **lubricant,** preferably a water-based jelly, to cover the penis before gently inserting it into the anus. Lubricants, such as K-Y Jelly, can be purchased over-the-counter at most drug stores.

Couples should never have vaginal intercourse after anal intercourse, because the penis is likely to contain bacteria. If it is placed inside the vagina after anal intercourse, a woman is likely to get a serious vaginal infection. Washing the penis with soap and warm water after anal sex is important.

Another risky behavior is **analingus,** commonly referred to as "rimming." Analingus is the oral stimulation, or licking, of the anal regions. By placing one's mouth on someone's anal area, a person is at risk for various infections and STDs.

VAGINAL INTERCOURSE

Vaginal intercourse is the insertion of the penis into the vagina. It is also called sex, coitus, and intercourse. Risks associated with vaginal intercourse include pregnancy and STDs. Some women experience a **yeast infection** after having vaginal sex. A yeast infection is a vaginal infection due to an overgrowth of yeast that causes an unpleasant odor, itching or burning, and a discharge. Most yeast infections are not sexually transmitted, but trichomoniasis is. Women can get the infection by having sex without a condom with someone who is infected. Trichomoniasis can be treated with antibiotic pills. Two sexually transmitted diseases, chlamydia and gonorrhea, can also cause vaginal discharge and sometimes that discharge is the only symptom. Both can be treated with antibiotic shots or pills.

Fact Or Fiction?

Is lotion a good lubricant?

The Facts: Lotions and petroleum jellies can promote vaginal infections. Because these lubricants are not water-based, they can break down a condom, reducing protection from pregnancy and STDs. If a woman's vagina is not lubricated or wet enough for intercourse, she can use a water-based lubricant such as K-Y Jelly. Water-based lubricants are sold at most drug stores. Some people use their saliva as a lubricant.

TEENS SPEAK

Saying "No" to My Boyfriend

My boyfriend and I had been dating for about three months. He kept pressuring me to have sex with him. I just didn't think I was ready. I'm only 15 and want to stay a virgin for a while. One night before we started making out, I asked him if he was upset we hadn't had sex yet. He said, "I'm not upset because I care about you. But I'd like to take our relationship to the next level and have sex."

At that point I felt really nervous. I care about him too. I don't want to say no to him, just no to sex. I told him I wasn't ready yet. I said I really care about him and want to continue to be intimate, just not go all the way.

At first he seemed disappointed. But after we talked for a while, he understood and said he would wait. I now know he is special and will wait until I'm ready. I care for him even more now because of that.

AUTOEROTIC BEHAVIOR

Autoerotic behaviors include erotic dreams or fantasies that some people find sexually exciting. These experiences arise from one's imagination, life experiences, books, pictures, or movies.

Erotic dreams occur during sleep without conscious control. According to the Kinsey reports of 1948 and 1953—the largest study ever conducted on human sexual behavior—almost all males and two-thirds of females reported erotic dreams. A person may become sexually aroused and awaken during an erotic dream. **Orgasm** can also occur at this time. An orgasm is pleasurable, rhythmic muscle contractions in the genital area. Having an orgasm in one's sleep is called a **nocturnal emission**. Some people may refer to it as a "wet dream."

Fantasies can occur during masturbation, sexual activity, or daydreams. Fantasies occur when people think about things that sexually excite them. Like erotic dreams, fantasies are normal. Some people experience them, and others do not. What a person fantasizes about depends on the person.

OTHER SEXUAL BEHAVIORS

There are other ways people express sexuality. Some of these activities may seem unusual. Some are illegal. Although they may not be as common, they do happen. These activities range from group sex and cross-dressing to fetishisms and sadomasochism.

Group sex

Group sex refers to sexual activities that involve three or more people. Group sex can be riskier than having sex with one person. Having sex with different people at the same time increases the risk of getting an STD. Participants also put themselves and others at risk of emotional damage. People may get jealous or feel hurt later, knowing their partner was with someone else.

Cross-dressing

Cross-dressing involves wearing clothing associated with the opposite sex. Wearing these clothes in public is sexually arousing for some people, while others do so only in the privacy of their own homes. For example, a man may find it exciting to wear women's panties or a bra.

Sadomasochism

Sadomasochism, also known as S and M, involves expressing one's sexuality with pain. Sadists become sexually aroused by hurting their partners. Masochists find pain sexually exciting. Aggressive sexual behavior can include "love bites" or being whipped, bound, or spanked. Pain can range from very mild to severe. Bondage, or being tied up, is a form of S and M. Some forms of sadomasochism can be physically dangerous—even deadly.

Fetishism

A fetish is an obsessive fixation on an object or part of the body. Someone who has a fetish may be sexually aroused by underwear, a foot, a breast, hair. For the most part, a fetish does not hurt others.

Only rarely does it develop into something that might harm another. A fetish may become risky if a person with a fetish steals a particular object, such as someone's shoes or panties.

Exhibitionism
The sexual behaviors discussed so far are done alone or with the consent of another person. Some forms of sexual behavior are illegal, because the person doing them does not have the consent of his or her partner. Victims of such acts may feel traumatized and violated. They may also feel vulnerable.

One potentially harmful behavior is **exhibitionism,** often called "indecent exposure." A person, usually male, shows or flashes his genitals publicly.

Exhibitionists gain sexual gratification without becoming emotionally connected or involved in a relationship. They flash to get a response. They are hoping that others will react in shock, fear, terror, or disgust. Since they are looking for a reaction, people shouldn't give them one. Exhibitionists should be reported to the police, since the act is illegal.

Obscene phone calls
People who make obscene phone calls are similar to exhibitionists. They both not only feel inadequate and insecure but also have anxieties or stresses about sexual relationships. They experience arousal when they hear shock or fear in their victim's voice. Some may masturbate after hearing a shocked response. Most people who make obscene phone calls are male.

The best way to handle an obscene phone call is to hang up the phone. The caller probably selected the phone number at random and does not know whom he is calling. If the phone rings again, ignore it. If the caller is persistent, take additional steps by blowing a loud whistle into the phone when he rings again, tracing the call, calling the police, or changing the phone number.

Voyeurism
Voyeurism is yet another illegal sexual behavior. Voyeurs get sexual satisfaction from watching a person without his or her consent. These people are also known as "peeping Toms." Voyeurs sometimes peek into someone's window to watch him or her in the shower or drill

holes into a wall to spy on the object of their interest. Voyeurs may also set up video cameras to record others without their knowledge. Males who are anxious or stressed about sexual relationships are most likely to become voyeurs. They seem to feel power over the individuals that they secretly observe. It is important to report voyeurs to the police as soon as possible.

VARIATIONS IN SEXUAL EXPRESSION

People express sexuality in a variety of ways. Sexual expression is different for each person. Ways of expressing sexuality range from celibacy to autoerotic behaviors. Any behaviors that are illegal and could be harmful or hurtful to other should be avoided. Couples should discuss their preferences and engage only in sexual activities that are comfortable for both partners.

See also: Basics of Gender Identity; Sexual Orientation

FURTHER READING

Abbott, Elizabeth. *A History of Celibacy: From Athena to Elizabeth I, Leonardo da Vinci, Florence Nightingale, Gandhi, and Cher.* New York: Scribner, 2000.

Bullough, Vern, and Bonnie Bullough. *Cross Dressing, Sex and Gender.* Philadelphia: University of Pennsylvania Press, 1993.

Lips, Hilary. *Sex and Gender.* 4th ed. Mountain View, Calif.: Mayfield, 2001.

■ SEXUAL ORIENTATION

An enduring emotional, romantic, or sexual attraction to another person. Those who are attracted to people of the opposite gender are considered **heterosexual.** Those who are attracted to people of their own gender are considered **homosexual.** Persons with a homosexual orientation are sometimes referred to as "gay" (both men and women) or "lesbian" (women only). Some people are attracted to both their own and the opposite sex. They are considered **bisexual.** Human beings do not choose their sexual orientation. For most people it emerges in early adolescence without prior sexual experience.

DID YOU KNOW?

How People Identify Their Sexual Orientation

	Men	Women
Identify self as homosexual	2.3%	1.4%
Had a sexual experience with the same sex	3.0%	4.0%
Have feelings of attraction toward someone of the same sex	4.1%	4.0%

Source: CDC: National Survey of Family Growth, 2002.

WHAT DETERMINES SEXUAL ORIENTATION?

Most experts believe that sexual orientation is a combination of what they refer to as **nature** and **nurture**. The word *nature* refers to biological factors like hormone levels, the brain, and genetics. *Nurture* describes psychosocial factors such as life experiences, childhood experiences, and psychological characteristics.

Spending time with someone who is gay will not cause a person to become homosexual. Not even engaging in sexual activity with a person of the same gender will cause a person to become gay. Some people experiment with their sexuality by engaging in sexual activities with people of the same gender. This behavior does not determine their sexual orientation. Sexual orientation refers to feelings rather than behaviors. People may or may not express their orientation through their actions.

COMING OUT

The term *coming out* describes the moment when a homosexual openly expresses his or her sexual orientation. The process begins with an acknowledgment of one's sexual orientation and an acceptance of it. Some people prefer to remain **in the closet**. They choose not to share their sexual preferences with others. Others remain in the closet because they fear that their friends or family will not be supportive.

Many gays suggest waiting to "come out" until one is sure he or she has the support of a few friends or family members. Coming out to one's parents can be particularly difficult. Some parents initially react with anger. The anger stems from feelings of guilt. They wonder what they did wrong. In fact, they did nothing wrong. No one is responsible for another person's sexual orientation.

Many parents learn to accept their child's sexual orientation. Others are supportive from the beginning. Almost all parents want their children to be happy whether they are heterosexual or homosexual. The same is true of friends. Some may respond with anger or surprise, but true friends will remain loyal regardless of one's sexual orientation.

TEENS SPEAK

Morgan Comes Out

Northern Seattle, where I'm from, is a pretty tolerant place. I go to an independent school that celebrates diversity, so when it came to telling my parents that I'm gay, I think I had it pretty easy. There was a lot of support from counselors and friend at school. Plus, my mom is a hairdresser. Her boss and a few of her coworkers are gay, and I've known them most of my life.

But even though there weren't any serious problems, it was still pretty stressful. I came out to my friends at school when I was 14, but I still hadn't told my parents. It felt like living a double life for awhile. I had to watch what I said. I stopped talking to my parents most of the time, and they started to seem like strangers. When my schoolwork started to suffer, I decided that was enough.

Mom didn't believe me at first. I think she was disappointed. My dad thought it was just a phase. He kept trying to point out attractive girls, hoping maybe that one would catch my eye and change my mind. I eventually had to tell him "Sorry, I just don't like girls." It's not just a phase. But I think he gets that now, and we talk again just like we used to.

CHANGING ATTITUDES TOWARD HOMOSEXUALITY

Early in the nation's history, many Americans regarded homosexuality as a sin. They were convinced that sexual activity between individuals of the same sex was evil, because they believed that the purpose of sexual activity was **reproduction,** producing offspring.

By the early to mid 1900s, attitudes toward gays began to change. Many people, including members of the American Psychiatric Association, now considered homosexuality a "sickness" rather than a sin. In their view, one's sexual orientation was a matter of choice. Choosing homosexuality indicated a mental disorder. It was not until 1973 that the American Psychiatric Association removed homosexuality from its list of mental disorders.

The change in attitude was prompted in part by **gay activists—** individuals who demanded rights for homosexuals. Inspired by the civil rights and women's rights movements of the 1960s, these men and women insisted on respect and equal rights. The turning point in gay and lesbian activism began during the weekend of June 27–29, 1969. On the night of the 27th, New York City police officers raided a dance bar called the Stonewall Inn in Greenwich Village. The excuse was the illegal sale of liquor, but the raid was part of a pattern of harassment gay bars experienced throughout the city in those days. That night, however, the routine raid quickly escalated into a riot.

Over the course of several days, gays and lesbians from all parts of the city fought back. In doing so, they changed the way homosexuals saw themselves and the way other Americans viewed gays and lesbians. The Stonewall Incident sparked the formation of dozens of gay rights groups, not only in New York but also in cities across the country.

A major goal of the new gay rights movement was the elimination of **sodomy laws** (laws that make oral and anal sex between consenting adults illegal). In 1969, every state had an antisodomy law. Some banned sodomy only between partners of the same sex. Others banned sodomy for everyone. Over the years, gay rights activists and others challenged those laws in state and federal courts. Little by little, those laws were repealed or blocked by state courts in 37 states.

In November 2003, the U.S. Supreme Court overturned Texas's sodomy law and in doing so declared similar laws in 12 other states unconstitutional. Justice Anthony Kennedy wrote for the court's majority, "The petitioners are entitled to respect for their private lives. The state cannot demean their existence or control their destiny by making their private sexual conduct a crime."

The gay rights movement has also tried to end discrimination based on sexual orientation by calling on state and federal governments to recognize crimes against gay men and women as hate crimes. At present, most state legislatures define a hate crime as the use of force or the threat of force to willfully injure, intimidate, interfere with, oppress, or threaten an individual because of his or her actual or perceived race, color, religion, ethnicity, or gender. Some also include crimes committed against individuals because of a physical or mental disability. Only a few mention sexual orientation. Gay activists would like sexual orientation included in the definitions of a hate crime throughout the nation.

Currently, the debate over the rights of gays and lesbians is focused on same-sex marriages. Some people oppose these marriages, because they view marriage solely as a union between a man and a woman. Those who support same-sex marriage believe two people in a committed relationship, regardless of their sexual orientation, should be able to marry. Other Americans favor a **civil union** for same-sex couples, or a legal recognition of their relationship. Such recognition would entitle their partners to many of the same benefits that spouses enjoy in traditional marriages—including adoption rights and rights to pension plans and health insurance coverage.

Q & A

Question: Why should heterosexuals support the rights of homosexuals?

Answer: In supporting gay rights, heterosexuals are supporting their own rights as well. If governments can deny people their rights because they are gay or bisexual, they can also deny the rights of other groups. One way heterosexuals can support homosexuals is to supporting groups that work for gay rights. Another way is by speaking out when friends make hateful comments or hurtful jokes about homosexuals.

SOCIETAL ATTITUDES TOWARD SEXUAL ORIENTATION

As people learn more about sexual orientation, they tend to become more tolerant of sexual preferences that differ from their own. For the first time, many people are seeing homosexuals portrayed positively in the media. A new gay and lesbian network on TV, Logo, brings stories and shows to the public that wouldn't be seen anywhere else.

Some people have intense but irrational fears of and strong prejudices against homosexuals. These people are described as being **homophobic.** These negative attitudes are expressed in aggression toward homosexuals, rude comments, or making fun of them. A 2008 Gallup poll revealed that Americans are evenly divided over the morality of homosexual relations, with 48 percent considering them morally acceptable and 48 percent saying they are morally wrong.

Support for the legality of homosexual relations has advanced and receded over the years, beginning at 43 percent when Gallup first asked about it in 1977. Support then dipped in the 1980s to the low 30s, but gradually increased through the 1990s and reached 60 percent in May 2003.

The critical issue for the gay rights movement today is same-sex marriage. The latest poll shows there is still considerable public resistance to giving the same legal sanction to same-sex couples as the law does to traditional marriages. As Gallup reported in 2008, only 40 percent of Americans say such marriages should be legally valid, as they now are in Massachusetts, Connecticut, Iowa, and Vermont, while 56 percent disagree.

TEENS SPEAK

Stop the Hate

I am a 16-year-old male who is tired of being discriminated against because of my sexual orientation. People always make fun of me and call me names like "fag," "homo," and "gay." They also say hateful things, like telling me that I am wrong. I kind of got used to it, but that's not right. I'm not supposed to get used to it. I'm supposed to stop it, but how? People can be so mean. My friends stick up for me, but I just take it. I hate it, but what can I do? To top it off, even parents say stuff to me! Why can't I be who I am without being hated?

VARIATIONS IN SEXUAL ORIENTATION

One's sexual orientation—whether heterosexual, homosexual, or bisexual—is a part of one's identity. Sexual orientation is not something a person chooses or can change. Being supportive of people regardless of their sexual orientation leads to a more accepting and supportive society.

See also: Sexual Arousal; Sexual Expression

■ SEXUAL PREDATORS

A name commonly applied to someone who commits sex crimes, such as rape or the sexual abuse of children. The term does not necessarily denote criminal behavior, however. Someone trying to find a sex partner in a predatory manner is also called a sexual predator. These people are not looking for fulfilling relationships but rather the gratification of their urges.

Many times the term sexual predator and **sexual offender** are used interchangeably, but a sexual offender is a person who has committed a sex crime, such as assault, indecent exposure, or rape. The term *sexual predator* is often used to refer to a person who has a habit of seeking sexual satisfaction at the emotional and physical expense of others.

PEDOPHILIA

Pedophilia involves sexual attraction toward children and usually involves males. Pedophilia is very rare among females. It is characterized by reoccurring, intense sexually arousing fantasies, sexual urges, or behaviors involving sexual activity with a child or children. According to the National Registry of Sex Officers, four percent of the population suffers from sexual orientation toward children.

A variety of different theories exist trying to explain the causes of pedophilia. A few researchers attribute pedophilia to biology. They hold that testosterone, one of the male sex hormones, predisposes men to develop deviant sexual behaviors. Pedophilia seems to be caused by a combination of genetic and environmental factors. Pedophiles are very likely to have been victims of sexual abuse as children.

Fact Or Fiction?

Sex crimes are crimes of passion or desire.

The Facts: Every sex crime is a crime of violence, anger, and power. These crimes are about controlling the victim. In cases of stranger rape, victims are often chosen based on vulnerability, not physical appearance.

Rates of Child Sexual Abuse

83,000 children were sexually abused in 2005.
906,000 children are victims of abuse yearly.
40 percent of children were molested by family members.

Source: Darkness to Light. URL: http://www.darkness2light.org, 2008.

According to the Child Molestation Research and Prevention Institute, it is estimated that at least two out of every 10 girls and one out of every 10 boys are sexually abused by the age of 13. The abusers who commit 95 percent of the sex acts against children are driven by an ongoing sex drive directed toward children. An estimated one in 20 teenage boys and adult men sexually abuse children, and an estimated one teenage girl or adult woman in every 3,300 females molests children. Add together the child victims, the adult survivors, and the abusers, and that is 15 out of every 100 Americans who have been either a molested child or a molester. Experts recommend that children be taught to yell or run if they are faced with an uncomfortable situation. They should also be taught that it is acceptable to scream or call for help in such situations.

CHILD PORNOGRAPHY

An image, video, or other form of **pornography** that involves children is child pornography. The possession or distribution of child pornography is illegal under federal laws in all 50 states. It is important to realize that these images can have a devastating and lasting effect on children. In addition to any physical injuries they can suffer in the course of their molestation, child victims can also experience depression, withdrawal, anger, and other psychological disorders. Such effects may continue into adulthood.

Almost all child pornography possessors arrested between July 1, 2000, and June 30, 2001—an estimated 1,713 people—were male, 91 percent were white, and 86 percent were older than 25. Only 3 percent were younger than 18. Most were unmarried at the time of their crime, either because they had never married (41 percent) or because they were separated, divorced, or widowed (21 percent). Thirty-eight percent were either married or living with partners.

Child victims also frequently experience feelings of guilt and responsibility for the abuse. The U.S. Department of Justice created the Child Exploitation and Obscenity Section in 1987 to protect children and communities by enforcing laws relating to the exploitation of children and obscenity.

Fact Or Fiction?

Sexual offenders commit these crimes in order to get sex.

The Facts: Sex offenders get gratification from intimidating, humiliating, and degrading their victims. Many sex offenders are married or already involved in relationships where they can freely engage in intimate relations, so it is not a lack of sex that drives them to commit these crimes.

INTERNET PREDATORS

An **Internet predator** is an Internet user who exploits vulnerable people online, usually for sexual or financial purposes. Most Internet sex offenders are young adults who target younger people. Adolescents and the elderly are most often the victims of online predators.

In a 2000 study, the National Center for Missing and Exploited Children and the Justice Department said that one of every five young people ages 10 to 17 surveyed said they had received a sexual solicitation over the Internet in the previous year. One in four teen girls in the United States reported that they met strangers off the Internet. One in seven boys admitted they did as well. While most of these "Internet friends" turn out to be another teen or preteen, that's not always the case. Individuals looking for potential child victims online have no difficulty finding them. It is quite common for these offenders to frequent "kids only" chat rooms and communicate with children who unwittingly divulge personal information about themselves. The result of these chats is sometimes the solicitation of sex over the Internet. Encounters with Internet predators can even be deadly.

Fact Or Fiction?

It's easy to tell who is a sex offender.

The Facts: Sex offenders come from all walks of life and ethnic backgrounds. A sex offender can be anyone: male, female, married, a friend, relative, acquaintance, or stranger. Sex offenders may even look "wholesome" or possess "movie star" good looks, which they use to make their approach to victims easier.

SEX OFFENDER REGISTRY

On March 5, 2003, the Supreme Court ruled that information about registered sex offenders may be posted on the Internet. The Dru Sjodin National Sex Offender Public Web Site is offered by the U.S. Department of Justice. People can view information about all registered sex offenders in the area, including how close the offenders reside to people's homes and children. In May 1996 Megan's Law was created, and it mandates that every state notify people where sex offenders live. This law was named after seven-year-old Megan Kanka, who was lured by her neighbor, a two-time registered sex offender, and was raped, strangled, and killed.

In accordance with Megan's Law and the Jacob Wetterling Act, all 50 states are required to register sex offenders and perform community notification. However, each state differs in terms of how it administers its community notification process, what offenders are required to register, the duration of registration, what information is registered, how the information is shared, whether the public has access to the registry, who is granted access, which methods of access are available, what information is shared—and that's just for starters.

PROTECTING YOURSELF

Experts recommend the following precautions: Be alert to your surroundings and trust your instincts. If you feel uncomfortable about a person or a location, leave immediately. Always know your location. If you must call 911, the operator must know the exact location of the emergency. Know your neighborhood: Where is the nearest police precinct? Which stores, restaurants, or businesses are open late at night? Where are public telephones located?

Learn to notice details about people. This will help you to give a good description. Take note of a person's coloring, size, hairstyle, facial hair, scars, tattoos, teeth, accent, and clothing.

Young adults should trust their instincts when they are with someone that makes them feel uncomfortable (e.g., in an elevator, in a car, in your home). This can be especially difficult for both children and adults who have been socialized to be polite. Do not talk yourself out of feeling uncomfortable when alone with someone simply because he or she is an acquaintance or a friend of a friend—most sexual abusers are someone the victim knows. Be wary of friends or dates that test your boundaries by making unwanted physical advances to you and then ignore or minimize your protests.

See Also: Violence, Sexual

FURTHER READING
Child Exploitation and Obscenity Section of the U.S. Department of Justice Web site. URL: http://www.justice.gov/criminal/ceos. Accessed February 24, 2009.
Darkness to Light Web site. URL: http://darkness2light.org. Accessed February 24, 2009.
Dru Sjodin National Sex Offender Public Web site. URL: http://www. nsopr.gov. Accessed February 24, 2009.

■ SEXUAL RESPONSE
Physical changes characteristic of healthy functioning that occur in the body as a result of sexual activity. The **sexual response cycle** describes the physical changes that take place during sexual arousal and activity. The cycle can be roughly divided into four phases, even though each person may experience these phases differently.

THE SEXUAL RESPONSE CYCLE
The sexual response cycle consists of four phases that both men and women may experience when they have sex. The phases are desire, excitement, orgasm, and resolution. Although each phase is experienced in that order, the cycle can be disrupted at any

phase. Not everyone reaches orgasm each time sexual excitement occurs.

Desire is essentially a longing or yearning to participate in sexual activity. It may begin with thoughts about sex or an attraction to another person. From the teenage years on, sexual desire is a part of life.

Desire can be stimulated by sight, sound, smell, touch, taste, movement, fantasy, and memory. Each can create a strong yearning for sexual stimulation (either by oneself or with another person) or sexual intimacy. What a person considers sexual or attractive varies greatly by culture and personal preference based on his or her thoughts, feelings, and experiences.

The second phase, **excitement,** is the feeling of arousal or being "turned on." The excitement may be the result of a sexual fantasy, erotic sights, sounds, scents, tastes, or touch. Physically, excitement means that the heart beats faster, blood pressure increases, and breathing becomes heavier. In both men and women, blood is sent to the genital area. Men experience an erection, or a stiff penis, and women lubrication or moistness in their vagina, which slightly increases in size. In both males and females, the skin of the genitals turns a deeper color.

The progression from desire to excitement depends on a variety of factors. For some people, particularly for some adolescents, the excitement stage requires very little physical or mental stimulation. For others, it may require physical stimulation or fantasy. It generally takes longer for women to achieve full arousal than for men to do so.

Orgasm, the third phase, is sexual climax. Orgasm occurs when the muscles around the genitals contract in rhythm, sending waves of pleasurable feelings through the body. In men, these muscle contractions cause semen to be ejaculated. Many women cannot reach orgasm from intercourse alone. They also need to experience stimulation to the **clitoris,** the external organ located above the vagina that is the center of arousal in females.

In the fourth phase, **resolution,** the body returns to the unexcited state. Mental excitement decreases, blood drains from the genital areas, and heartbeat and breathing slow. Resolution occurs a few minutes after an orgasm. Even if a person does not reach orgasm, resolution still takes place, but more slowly. Although not reaching orgasm may be frustrating, it is not harmful. Some men and women experience a minor ache until the extra blood leaves the genital area.

Fact Or Fiction?

My girlfriend and I should both orgasm at the same time.

The Facts: Although possible, it is unlikely that two people will reach orgasm at the same time, since they each experience the stages of the sexual response cycle differently. One person may not be ready for the orgasm stage as soon as the other person is. It is most common for one person to orgasm first.

CONCERNS FOR MEN

Males have specific issues in regard to the sexual response cycle. Unlike women, men have a **refractory period,** a time after an orgasm in which they are not physically capable of having another orgasm. As a man ages, this period gets longer. A man in his seventies may need to wait several days before having another erection. A man in his late teens or early twenties may only need to wait a few minutes.

Men may also experience **impotence,** the inability to achieve an erection. Impotence is a common problem usually arising from the use of drugs or alcohol or a psychological problem. It can also be caused by medical conditions, such as diabetes or blood vessel diseases. Men may need help from a physician or counselor, although sometimes just talking with their partner can help.

Another concern is **premature ejaculation,** or ejaculating too quickly when stimulated and excited. With time, men can learn to control their ejaculation. However, premature ejaculation can be a problem for teens if they are using **withdrawal,** or the removal of the penis from the vagina before ejaculating, to prevent pregnancy.

Men may also feel pressure to "perform" well. Many falsely believe that they are judged on their "performance" or "accomplishment." Some feel that their partner expects them to help her reach orgasm or wait to have an orgasm until she has done so. It is important for men to talk to their partners and communicate openly about what each person wants.

Q & A

Question: What is erectile dysfunction and what causes it?

Answer: Medical problems can cause impotence or erectile dysfunction including diabetes (high blood sugar), hypertension (high blood pressure), and atherosclerosis (hardening of the arteries). Erectile dysfunction may also be the result of a hormonal imbalance. Some medicines can also cause the problem. Consuming too much alcohol, nicotine, or illegal drugs can also result in impotence. Sometimes the problem is not medical. Difficulties with a sexual partner also can cause erectile dysfunction.

CONCERNS FOR WOMEN

Unlike men, women do not need a refractory period before having another orgasm. However, **anorgasmia,** the inability to reach an orgasm, is more common among women than men. Fatigue, stress, feeling pressured to have sex, or, perhaps, having a sexual partner who is not aware of a woman's needs may lead to anorgasmia. A woman who has been raped may become unable to enjoy sex. A woman's values and beliefs about sex may also increase anorgasmia. In some cultures, women are not supposed to enjoy or be interested in sex.

Other concerns for women include dyspareunia and vaginismus. Dyspareunia is mild to severe pain during sex. The pain may be a result of hormonal imbalances, sexual inhibitions, or a poor relationship with a partner. If the use of lubricants and longer stimulation do not relieve the symptoms, the woman should consult her physician.

Vaginismus is an involuntary spasm of the muscles around the vagina, making penetration difficult and painful, or even impossible. A woman with vaginismus may experience great pain when attempting intercourse with her partner. She may even find it painful to insert a tampon. Vaginismus may be the result of a conditioned response that reflects fear, anxiety, or pain due to negative attitudes about sex, sexual abuse, or negative early sexual experiences.

Many people, men and women alike, experience sexual difficulty at some point in their lives, and there is no shame in seeking help or advice.

RESPONDING SEXUALLY

For some, sex is a pleasurable experience, while for others it is not. Although the sexual response cycle prepares the body for pleasure leading to orgasm, not everyone experiences orgasm. Some may even suffer pain or discomfort with sexual activity. When two people are sexually active and want to enjoy a sexual relationship, knowing each other's needs is important.

See also: Biology and Sex; Sexual Arousal

■ SEXUALLY TRANSMITTED DISEASES (STDs)

More than 20 different types of infections may be passed from one person to another by sexual contact such as vaginal, anal, or oral sex, and possibly by wet kissing. Some sexually transmitted diseases (STDs) cause pain and discomfort, embarrassment, emotional problems, **infertility** (the inability to conceive a child), and even death. Many bacterial STDs can be successfully treated with antibiotics. Viral STDs, however, have no cure.

DANGERS OF UNPROTECTED SEX

Teens have choices about their relationships and how far they are willing to go. With these choices come responsibilities. Teens who are sexually active have responsibilities to themselves and their partners. Those responsibilities include honesty about medical conditions that could affect a partner.

Some STDs cannot be successfully treated at this time. A person could have these diseases for life. Although there are treatments to reduce the symptoms, the disease remains in the body. Those who have the disease are contagious for life and can pass it on to future partners. Having unprotected sex even once can result in a lifelong disease. If a person suspects he or she has been exposed to an STD, the best thing to do is to get tested.

Q & A

Question: How do I get tested for an STD?

Answer: Most health clinics or health departments offer free or inexpensive testing. Testing is also available from Planned Parenthood. Most clinics offer a variety of tests, because different STDs require different tests. There is no one test that can be used to detect every STD.

In testing for chlamydia or gonorrhea, a long cotton swab is used to gather a small amount of fluid from inside the penis or the vagina near the cervix. When a physician examines the fluid, he or she looks for the bacterium that causes chlamydia or gonorrhea. Testing for herpes or genital warts requires a visual exam. If no sores are present, the physician may order a blood test. A blood test may also be used to test for HIV.

HOW COMMON ARE STDS IN TEENS?

Teens have the highest rates of STDs in the nation. In 2003, according to the Centers for Disease Control and Prevention's (CDC's) Division of Sexually Transmitted Diseases, one in four sexually active teen girls

DID YOU KNOW?

Annual Number of STD Cases in the United States in 2005

STD	Est. Annual Number of Cases
Genital Warts (HPV)	6.2 million
Trichomoniasis	7.4 million
Chlamydia	3 million
Herpes	1 million
Gonorrhea	700,000
Hepatitis B	77,000
Syphilis	70,000
HIV/AIDs	45,669

Source: American Social Health Association, 2005.

was infected with an STD at any given time. In 2007, the CDC estimated that approximately 19 million new infections occur each year. Almost half of them are young people 15 to 24 years of age. These numbers may seem surprising, because STDs are not frequently discussed. Many people are embarrassed, uncomfortable, or lack the necessary information to talk about sexually transmitted diseases publicly.

HOW TO PREVENT STDS

The best way to protect oneself from an STD is **abstinence,** or choosing not to have sex. For those who are sexually active, a condom provides the best protection against sexually transmitted diseases. Those who claim condoms are uncomfortable or too much trouble should keep in mind that many STDs are even more uncomfortable. They can also be painful and can last for life. The following suggestions are ways of protecting oneself against STDs:

- Choose abstinence.
- If you choose to have sex, always use a condom.
- Ask a partner if he or she has ever had an STD. Talk about STDs.
- Be in a **monogamous** relationship—one in which both partners are sexually active only with each other.
- Get tested before having sex and ask your partner to do the same.

Fact Or Fiction?

You can't get an STD if you wear a condom.

The Facts: Condoms are designed to prevent the exchange of bodily fluids. They protect people from many STDs that are present in vaginal fluid and semen, such as HIV, gonorrhea, and chlamydia. However, other STDs, such as herpes and genital warts, are transmitted by skin-to-contact and may be present in areas the condom doesn't cover, such as the testicles, the inner thighs, or the anus.

Q & A

Question: Can I get an STD if I don't have sex?

Answer: A person can get STDs such as gonorrhea and herpes through oral sex. Gonorrhea produces a sore throat and pus, or discharge. **Oral herpes,** commonly referred to as cold sores, is easily transmitted by kissing or by sharing food and drink with someone who has oral herpes.

VIRAL STDS

Those who have a **viral STD,** such as herpes, genital warts, hepatitis B, or HIV, have a disease for which there is no cure. They are likely to have the virus in their body for life. Viral STDs do not respond to antibiotics. Most people with these STDs do not always have symptoms and some never have any. Yet a person with a viral STD, whether he or she has a single symptom, can spread the disease to others. When symptoms do appear, doctors usually prescribe an antiviral medicine.

Most people with a viral STD have few or no symptoms until the STD reaches a dangerous stage, the stage at which the STD can affect a person's **fertility**—a female's ability to produce healthy eggs and a male's ability to produce sperm for reproduction.

STDs become dangerous in women when they travel beyond the **cervix,** the opening to the uterus located at the top of the **vagina,** to the **fallopian tubes.** The vagina is the birth canal. The fallopian tubes are where **fertilization,** the fusion of the egg and sperm, takes place.

In men, STDs become dangerous when they pass through the **urethra,** the passageway for urine and sperm, to the epididymis or the **testes.** The epididymis is the comma-shaped organ that lies along the back of the testes. It is where sperm mature until they are ejaculated. The testes are the paired male organs that produce sperm and male hormones.

Herpes

Herpes is a viral STD that causes small, painful, red bumps filled with fluid. They resemble blisters in that when they rupture, they form wet, open sores. A person with herpes is always at risk of passing it to someone else, even when no symptoms are present. However, a person is more likely to pass on the STD when he or she has open sores.

Some people with herpes never have an outbreak of bumps or blisters. Others may get an outbreak once a month. It depends on the strength of a person's **immune system,** the system in the body that fights infection. Getting enough sleep and eating a healthy diet will help to improve one's immune system, thereby reducing the number of herpes outbreaks.

There are many kinds of herpes. Oral herpes or herpes-1 causes sores on the mouth. This virus is very common. Genital herpes, also known as herpes-2, results in cold sores in the genital area. The American Social Health Association estimates that one in five Americans has genital herpes. It is so prevalent because many people do not know they have the virus and therefore pass it on unknowingly to their partners. Of the people who have genital herpes, about half never experience an outbreak. It may be frightening to realize that a person can get a virus, have no symptoms, and yet pass it to someone else.

HPV and genital warts

Genital warts (or condyloma) is an STD caused by the human papilloma virus (HPV). The virus can result in wartlike bumps on the penis, in and around the vagina, on the cervix, in the anus, and occasionally on the mouth. The virus is passed between people during anal, vaginal, and sometimes oral sex.

Scientists have identified more than 100 types of HPV. Although most types are harmless, more than 40 types are spread through sexual contact. Some types of HPV that cause genital infections can also cause cervical cancer and other genital cancers. Although the warts do not hurt, they can cause problems if they are not removed by a doctor. Like herpes, genital warts can be passed from one person to another even when there are no visible symptoms. Although a doctor can remove the warts, the virus remains in the body.

Females are at an increased risk of cervical cancer if they come in contact with certain strains of HPV. To test for cervical cancer, a woman should begin receiving a yearly **Pap smear** at age 21, or when she becomes sexually active.

Like many STDs, genital HPV infections often do not have visible signs and symptoms. One study sponsored by the National Institute of Allergy and Infectious Diseases (NIAID) reported that almost one-half of women infected with HPV had no obvious symptoms. People who are infected but who have no symptoms may not realize that they can transmit HPV to others or that they can develop complications from the virus.

According to the National Institutes of Health, the United States has more cases of genital HPV infection than of any other STD. Approximately 20 million people are currently infected. At least 50 percent of sexually active men and women acquire genital HPV infection at some point in their lives. By age 50, about 80 percent of women will have had a genital HPV infection. About 6.2 million Americans get a new genital HPV infection each year.

There is now a vaccine that prevents infection from the type of HPV that cause most cases of cervical cancer and genital warts. The vaccine, Gardasil, is given in three shots over six months. The vaccine is routinely recommended for 11- and 12-year-old girls. It is also recommended for girls and women age 13 through 26 who have not yet been vaccinated or completed the vaccine series. It is highly effective in preventing those types of HPV and related diseases in young women. Every year, about 12,000 women are diagnosed with cervical cancer and almost 4,000 women die from this disease in the United States.

Q & A

Question: How do I tell my partner I have an STD?

Answer: Tell your partner in a way that is comfortable for you. Many people prefer to do so privately and in person. Explain that you're not sure who had it first (if you haven't had any other partners) and that it really doesn't matter. What matters is that your partner gets tested and you both get treated to prevent the STD from getting worse.

BACTERIAL STDS

Bacterial STDs include chlamydia, gonorrhea, and syphilis. Chlamydia affects about four million Americans every year. It is particularly common among teenagers. Gonorrhea infects about 700,000 Americans each year, according to the CDC; syphilis, about 36,000 people.

If chlamydia and gonorrhea are not treated with antibiotics, they can lead to complications. Risks associated with these infections include infertility, **pelvic inflammatory disease** (PID), and cancer of the penis or cervix. PID is an infection of the fallopian tubes in which scar tissue may form within the tubes and block the passage of eggs and sperm, leading to infertility.

Syphilis is an easily curable STD. The disease proceeds in four stages as the bacteria make their way to various organs in the body. Although the early symptoms of syphilis are very mild, the disease is very contagious during these early stages. Later, when syphilis is no longer contagious, it can, if left untreated, cause serious heart abnormalities, mental disorders, blindness, and death.

The rate of syphilis in its early stages declined in the United States by 89.2 percent between 1990 and 2000. The number of new cases rose, however, from 5,979 in 2000 to 6,103 in 2001. According to the CDC, these were the first increases since 1990. The CDC reports the rate of syphilis has risen 12 percent between 2006 and 2007. The number of reported cases of syphilis increased from 9,756 in 2006 to 11,181 in 2007. The CDC attributes this increase to new cases of syphilis among gay and bisexual men. The increase is of particular concern because people in the early stages of syphilis are three to five times more susceptible to HIV, the virus that causes AIDS, than other people.

Although all bacterial STDs can be cured with antibiotics, many people with these diseases have no symptoms. When symptoms are present, males experience painful or burning urination and milky or puslike discharge from the penis. Females have a vaginal discharge, painful or frequent urination, and pain in the pelvic area. Since bacterial STDs can be cured with antibiotics, anyone who has ever had unprotected sex should be tested.

TEENS SPEAK

I Found Out I Have Chlamydia

I'm 15 and recently found out that I have chlamydia. I'm not even sure how I got it. I've only had sex with my boyfriend, who says he's only had sex with me and a girlfriend before me. I guess he got chlamydia and didn't know it.

I never thought this would happen to me. I'm a good student, involved in a few clubs, and play soccer. I don't feel sick. I didn't even have symptoms.

I only got tested because we talked about STDs in health class, and I learned how common they are. To my surprise,

I had chlamydia. Now what? At first I thought my life was over. Then, I found out it could be cured. I called the local county health department and talked to a great nurse over the phone. She told me everything I needed to know and helped me to get an antibiotic. I told my boyfriend and he was very supportive. He, too, got tested and got antibiotics to treat chlamydia. We also use a condom every time now.

Q & A

Question: Can pregnant women pass STDs to their unborn babies?

Answer: HIV and syphilis can cross the placenta, affecting the fetus while it is developing. Herpes, genital warts, chlamydia, and gonorrhea can affect the baby as it passes through the vagina during delivery. If the doctor knows the expectant mother has a sexually transmitted disease, he or she can take steps to prevent the STD from spreading to the baby. For example, recent government studies reveal that by treating infants exposed to HIV with drugs used to fight AIDS drugs, physicians can prevent the transmissions of AIDS from mother to child.

HIV AND AIDS

When someone is infected with HIV, his or her body tries to fight the infection by producing antibodies, special molecules that are supposed to fight the virus. When people have HIV, the virus attacks and takes over the cells that protect the body from infections. HIV slowly wears down the immune system. Once the immune system is damaged, viruses, parasites, fungi, and bacteria that usually don't cause people problems can make them very sick.

Being HIV-positive, or having HIV, is not the same as having AIDS. Many people are HIV-positive but don't get sick for many years. The average time it takes the HIV virus to become AIDS is about 10 years.

You cannot get HIV from a hug, a toilet, or an eating utensil used by someone with HIV. You can only get HIV by:

- Having unprotected sex;
- Sharing contaminated needles;

DID YOU KNOW?

Exposures Causing People to Get AIDS, 1998–2005

Exposure category	1998	1999	2000	2001	2002	2003	2005
Male adult or adolescent							
Male-to-male sexual contact	17,357	16,378	16,076	16,296	16,944	15,859	18,296
Injection drug use	8,462	7,965	7,689	7,115	6,945	4,866	3,441
Male-to-male sexual contact and injection drug use	2,466	2,275	2,006	2,010	1,898	1,695	1,324
Heterosexual contact	4,033	4,136	4,258	4,554	4,937	3,371	4,255
Other*	384	365	367	361	365	185	139
Subtotal	32,703	31,119	30,396	30,335	31,089	25,976	27,455
Female adult or adolescent							
Injection drug use	3,740	3,516	3,533	3,387	3,180	2,262	1,851
Heterosexual contact	6,300	6,260	6,911	7,103	7,476	5,234	7,734
Other*	243	236	281	292	299	119	124
Subtotal	10,283	10,012	10,725	10,783	10,955	7,615	9,709
Child ([greater than]13 yrs)							
Prenatal or postnatal	236	181	115	106	90	131	142
Other*	1	2	3	4	2	21	26
Subtotal	238	183	118	110	92	152	168

* Includes hemophilia and transfusions

Source: Centers for Disease Control and Prevention, 2005.

- Receiving contaminated blood from a blood transfusion; or
- Breast-feeding.

If a person has HIV, he or she may experience flulike symptoms at first. Later one may notice unexplained tiredness, weight loss, skin conditions, diarrhea, lung infections, or changes in one's mental state. Although no cure exists, many medicines are now available that reduce the symptoms and help people with HIV live longer. Support from family and friends is also important for someone who has HIV.

PROTECTING ONESELF

Since teens are the fastest growing group of people with STDs, protecting oneself is important. Abstinence is the only sure way to avoid sexually transmitted diseases. Those who are sexually active can protect themselves by using a condom every time they have sex and getting tested for STDs. Not everyone has symptoms when he or she has an STD, and many symptoms are too mild to notice.

See also: Contraceptives Involving Risk; Pelvic Inflammatory Disease; Violence, Sexual

FURTHER READING
Ciambrone, Desirée. *Women's Experiences with HIV/AIDS.* Binghamton, N.Y.: Haworth Press, 2003.
Klauser, Jeffrey. *Current Diagnosis and Treatment of Sexually Transmitted Diseases.* New York: McGraw Hill, 2007.
Smith, P. A. *Encyclopedia of AIDS: A Social, Cultural, and Scientific Study.* Cambridge, Mass.: Perseus, 2002.

■ VIOLENCE, SEXUAL

Forced sexual activity. Sexual violence can range from unwanted touching and grabbing to sexual intercourse.

Many states now use the term **sexual assault** to describe all forced sexual contact, including **rape**. Rape is forced sexual penetration. It is a crime in every state. Some states substitute the term *aggravated sexual assault* for *rape,* and many states include homosexual rape, incest (sexual intercourse between persons too closely related to marry, as between a parent and a child), and other sex offenses in the definition of rape.

SEXUAL ASSAULT

Sexual assault includes unwanted touching as well as penetration. If someone has been sexually assaulted, he or she may have been grabbed in an inappropriate way or forced to perform oral sex. According to the Department of Justice (DOJ), one in five females and one in 10 males will be sexually assaulted in their lifetime. Young boys are more likely to be victims of a sexual assault than older men.

Sexual violence is associated with aggression, abuse, and humiliation. People use sexual violence to harm, humiliate, or exploit others. Greater awareness and education may help to prevent sexual assaults or at least reduce the alarming numbers of victims in the United States.

A **perpetrator** is a person who commits an act of violence (in this case, a sexual assault). He or she may use brute force, drugs, alcohol, or verbal threats. People who commit acts of sexual violence do so to gain power and control over their **victim,** the person against whom the crime is committed. Perpetrators are not interested in sexual gratification. The motive is rarely sexual. Perpetrators are most often motivated by extreme anger toward the victim or a need to overpower him or her. Forced sex is intended to abuse, humiliate, and dehumanize the victim.

Sexual violence is never the fault of the victim. No one "deserves" to be sexually assaulted and no one ever "asks" for rape. Although females are more commonly the victims of sexual attacks, males may also be victims. Typically, the victim knows the perpetrator. Sexual assaults rarely involve strangers. In 2002 the Justice Department's National Crime Victimization Survey (NCVS) revealed that 70 percent of female victims and 67 percent of male victims knew the perpetrator of the crime. He or she was a spouse, friend, coworker, or date. These sexual assaults are known as **acquaintance rape** or date rape.

The National Institute of Justice (NIJ), the research and development agency of the DOJ, estimates that one million women are raped every year in the United States. Exact numbers are difficult to determine since many women do not report rape. The NIJ estimates that only 30 percent of all rapes are reported to the police, while 50 percent of the victims tell no one. Shame, fear of revenge or rejection, and fear of the trauma of a court trial are common reasons for the failure to report a sexual offense.

DID YOU KNOW?

Teens Raped in the United States in 2007

Grade	Percentage of teens who have been raped
Grade 9	6.6
Grade 10	8.2
Grade 11	8.5
Grade 12	8.3
Average, grades 9–12	7.8

Gender	Percentage of teens who have been raped
Males, grades 9-12	4.5
Females, grades 9-12	11.3

Source: Centers for Disease Control and Prevention, 2007.

Adolescent females and children make up the largest group of rape victims. Nearly one-half (44 percent) of all females who are victims of rape are under the age of 18 and 15 percent are under the age of 12. The term used to describe the rape of a person under the legal age of consent to sexual intercourse is **statutory rape**. States vary in defining the age of consent, but in most states, it ranges from 14 to 18 years of age.

Fact Or Fiction?

A girl who is drunk can still consent to sexual activity.

The Facts: A person who is drunk cannot legally consent to sex. Having sex with someone who is drunk or high on drugs is considered a sexual assault.

HOW COMMON IS SEXUAL ASSAULT?

Sexual assault is one of the most frequently committed violent crimes in the United States, according to the American College of Obstetricians and Gynecologists. Studies suggest that one in three women will be sexually assaulted in their lifetime. Men are also sexually assaulted. Some studies suggest as many as one in five males are sexually assaulted during their lifetime. From 1992 to 2000, the DOJ conducted the NCVS to determine the prevalence of sexual assault in the United States. The annual average number of rapes and sexual assaults was 366,460 for each year from 1994 to 2000. However, only 36 percent of these rapes and 26 percent of these rapes and sexual assaults were reported to police. In the same study, 94 percent of all rape victims, 91 percent of targets of attempted rapes, and 89 percent of all victims of completed and attempted sexual assaults were female.

Q & A

Question: How can I help a friend who has been the victim of sexual violence?

Answer: Your friend may experience many different emotional and physical reactions as a result of an assault, including:

- Loss of appetite. His or her interest in food may decrease or food may not taste right. Many people feel nauseous or have an upset stomach.

- Nightmares, difficulty getting to sleep, or waking up in the night and being unable to get back to sleep. Even a few days without a good night's sleep can increase stress levels. On the other hand, some people may sleep more than before.

- Depression. Many victims experience mood swings or crying spells. Though crying spells may be worrisome or frightening, they can also be a way to release tension.

- Difficulty making decisions that were easy to make before the assault. As a result of the assault, many things in the victim's life may feel out of control. That loss of control is part of the trauma of a sexual assault, and it takes most survivors time before they begin to feel in control of some things again.

Help your friend understand that his or her reactions are normal responses to a trauma. If your friend is eager to talk, listen. If your friend is reluctant to talk, understand that he or she may not be ready to express his or her feelings at this time. Give your friend space, but be there when he or she needs support. Remember that recovering from a sexual assault is hard. Having difficulty does not mean that he or she is mentally ill. Recovery takes time.

WHAT ARE THE EFFECTS OF SEXUAL VIOLENCE?

The long-term effects of sexual violence can be physically and emotionally hurtful. There is no specific pattern of response, since each person responds in his or her own way.

Initially, many victims experience shock, anxiety, or confusion. Denial is also common, especially among victims who have been assaulted by someone they know. As time passes, anger, shame, or guilt replace shock and anxiety. Social problems can sometimes occur following a sexual assault as well. The victim may have difficulty in maintaining or deepening relationships with friends, dating partners, or a spouse. Some lose interest in sexual activity.

A number of rape victims will experience what's known as **Rape Trauma Syndrome**, or RTS. RTS is a kind of psychological post-traumatic stress disorder, which often happens when people have potentially life-threatening experiences or are witness to other people having them. A person may experience different phases of RTS, and they may last weeks or years. Recovering from the experience of an assault may involve moving back and forth within these phases over the course of a lifetime.

After a rape, many women take **emergency contraception** (a pill to prevent pregnancy that is taken within 72 hours of unprotected sex). If a woman does become pregnant as the result of a rape, she may have to decide whether to seek an abortion. Another concern for both male and female victims is the possibility of acquiring a sexually transmitted disease (STD).

WHAT CAN A PERSON DO IF HE OR SHE IS SEXUALLY ASSAULTED?

Many people find it difficult to admit to being a victim, especially of a sexual assault. Victims should never be ashamed, since they did nothing wrong and are not at fault. After an assault, the victim should seek medical assistance as quickly as possible. A clinic or hospital can test not only for pregnancy or an STD but also treat and counsel victims. Just because a person seeks medical help doesn't mean that he or she has to press charges; that decision is up to the individual.

If a victim decides to press charges, it is best to do so as soon as possible. Going to the police early allows officers to collect physical evidence such as the perpetrator's body fluid, hair, and skin. Although many people want to shower after an assault, the water will wash away the evidence. Reporting the assault and telling the police the details may seem frightening, but it is the only way to stop the perpetrator from hurting someone else.

PROTECT YOURSELF AND OTHERS FROM SEXUAL ASSAULT

The following suggestions may lower the risk of a sexual assault:

- Travel in a group, especially when attending a party or social function. Be sure to keep track of each other and agree to leave together.

- Carry a cell phone or emergency cash for a phone call to a friend or parent or for cab fare. Do not hesitate to use it! Money can be hidden in a pocket, shoe, sock, bra, or small pouch pinned to the inside of your pants or skirt.

- If someone is bothering you, move to a crowded area. Don't hesitate to initiate a conversation with someone else as a way of getting rid of someone who is annoying you.

- Make eye contact and look at the person who seems to be following you or lurking by you. When someone feels they have been "seen," they are less likely to attack.

- Ask the person to stop following you or bothering you. Talking to the person shows you are assertive and may make him or her less likely to attack.

- Avoid alcohol, but if you drink, know your limits so you can control your decisions. According to the DOJ, 90 percent of all sexual assaults involve drugs or alcohol.

- Watch out for anyone who tries to get you drunk or puts some kind of drug in your glass. Throw away a drink you have left unattended.
- Keep your house, car door, etc., locked at all times.
- Communicate clearly. Tell someone if you do not want him or her to touch you.

CHILD SEXUAL ABUSE

More than 3.6 million cases of child abuse and neglect are reported each year in the United States, according to the American Academy of Pediatrics. About 9 percent involve sexual abuse. The National Center on Child Abuse and Neglect defines **child sexual abuse** as contacts between a child and an adult in which the child is being used for sexual stimulation of the adult or when the perpetrator is in a position of power or control over the victim.

Child sexual abuse includes not only physical contact, such as fondling or rape, but also forcing a child to watch sexual acts or **pornography** (a creative activity designed only to stimulate sexual desire), using a child to produce pornography, or making a child look at an adult's genitals.

Most sexual abusers are men, regardless of whether the victim is a boy or a girl. Women can also be perpetrators. Studies report that women commit 2 to 4 percent of reported sex offenses against children. Overall, 6 percent of offenders who sexually assaulted juveniles were female.

Most perpetrators know the child they abused but are not relatives. In fact, about 80 percent of all perpetrators are family friends, baby-sitters, or neighbors. About 30 percent are relatives of the child, such as fathers, uncles, or cousins. In just 10 percent of child sexual abuse cases, the perpetrator was a stranger. Many child pornographers and other perpetrators who are strangers make contact with children using the Internet.

How does one know if a child has been sexually abused? Obvious signs of abuse rarely exist. Although sexually abused children do exhibit some symptoms, there is rarely physical evidence. Child sexual abuse is also difficult to detect, because it usually occurs in private. Some children, however, may show signs of post-traumatic stress disorder, including agitated behavior, frightening dreams, and repetitive play in which aspects of the abuse are expressed. Children may also show sexual behavior or seductiveness that is inappropriate for their age.

As a result of abuse, some children, especially boys, tend to exhibit behavioral problems, such as cruelty to others and running away. Other children may become depressed or withdrawn. Still others may try to injure themselves or commit suicide.

The possible long-term effects of child sexual abuse include not only post-traumatic stress disorder, anxiety, and depression but also:

- Sexual anxiety and disorders;
- Poor body image and low self-esteem;
- Efforts to mask the painful emotions through alcohol abuse, drug abuse, self-mutilation, or bingeing and purging.

ENDING SEXUAL VIOLENCE

Knowing the risks of sexual violence and avoiding risky situations may help to protect potential victims. However, one cannot control the actions of perpetrators. Therefore, reporting sexual violence to the police is critical. Reporting sexual violence is the only way to prevent perpetrators from hurting someone else. In addition, talking about sexual violence and working towards ending this crime is necessary to better the lives of children, teens, and adults alike.

See also: Dating; Sex and the Law

FURTHER READING

Maltz, Wendy. *The Sexual Healing Journey.* New York: HarperCollins, 2001.

Venable Rain, Nancy. *After Silence: Rape and My Journey Back.* New York: Three Rivers Press/Crown, 1999.

Scarce, Michael. *Male on Male Rape.* New York: Plenum, 1997.

Schewe, P. A. *Preventing Violence in Relationships: Interviews across the Lifespan.* Washington, D.C.: American Psychological Association, 2002.

HOTLINES AND HELP SITES

American Social Health Association (ASHA)
URL: http://www.ashastd.org
Phone: (919) 361-8400
Address: American Social Health Association
  P.O. Box 13827
  Research Triangle Park, NC 27709
Affiliation: Nongovernmental resource
Mission: The American Social Health Association is dedicated to improving the health of individuals, families, and communities, with a focus on preventing sexually transmitted diseases (STDs) and their harmful consequences.
Programs: The American Social Health Association is recognized by the public, patients, providers and policymakers for developing and delivering accurate, medically reliable information about STDs. Public and college health clinics across the United States order ASHA educational pamphlets and books to give to clients and students. Community-based organizations depend on ASHA, too, to help communicate about risk, transmission, prevention, testing, and treatment.

CDC National STD, HIV/AIDS Hotline
Phone: (800) 227-8922 or (800) 342-2437
En español: (800) 344-7432
Hearing impaired: (800) 243-7889
Program: This hotline provides toll-free information on sexually transmitted diseases (STDs) and human immunodeficiency virus

(HIV) to the general public. Health communication specialists are trained to convey accurate, basic information and referrals to free or low-cost clinics nationwide. Free educational literature about a wide variety of STDs, including HIV, and prevention methods are also available. Service is available in English 24 hours per day, seven days a week; in Spanish, 8:00 A.M. until 2:00 A.M. ET, seven days a week; and via TTY for the deaf and hard of hearing, 10:00 A.M. until 10:00 P.M. ET, Monday through Friday.

Gender Identity Center of Colorado, The

URL: http://www.transgender.org/gic

Phone: (303) 202-6466

Address: 3895 Upham Street,

Suite 40

Wheat Ridge, CO 80033

E-mail: info@gicofcolo.org

Mission: This organization provides support and educational resources to people who are transsexual, cross-dress, or are otherwise nontraditional in their gender identity and/or behaviors.

Go Ask Alice!

URL: http://www.goaskalice.columbia.edu

Affiliation: *Go Ask Alice!* is the health question and answer Internet service produced by Alice!, Columbia University's Health Education Program, a division of Columbia University Health and Related Services.

Mission: The mission of *Go Ask Alice!* is to increase access to, and use of, health information by providing factual, in-depth, straightforward, and nonjudgmental information to assist readers' decision-making about their physical, sexual, emotional, and spiritual health.

Programs: Q&As of the Week gives you the latest inquiries and responses—this section is updated every Friday; Search GAA! lets you find health information by subject via a search of the ever-growing *Go Ask Alice!* archives, which contain 2,000 previously posted questions and answers; and Ask Alice! gives you the chance to ask Alice! a question.

Human Rights Campaign
URL: http://www.hrc.org
Phone: (202) 628-4160 or (800) 777-4723
TTY: (202) 216-1572
Address: 1640 Rhode Island Avenue, NW
  Washington, DC 20036-3278
Affiliation: Nonprofit organization
Mission: HRC is a bipartisan organization that works to advance equality based on sexual orientation and gender expression and identity, to ensure that gay, lesbian, bisexual and transgender Americans can be open, honest, and safe at home, at work, and in the community.
Programs: As America's largest gay and lesbian organization, the Human Rights Campaign provides a national voice on gay and lesbian issues. The Human Rights Campaign effectively lobbies Congress, mobilizes grassroots action in diverse communities, invests strategically to elect a fairminded Congress, and increases public understanding through innovative education and communication strategies.

Kinsey Institute for Research in Sex, Gender, and Reproduction
URL: http://www.kinseyinstitute.org
Affiliation: Founded in 1947, The Kinsey Institute for Research in Sex, Gender, and Reproduction is a private, not-for-profit corporation affiliated with Indiana University.
Mission: The mission of The Kinsey Institute is to promote interdisciplinary research and scholarship in the fields of human sexuality, gender, and reproduction.

Male Health Center
URL: http://www.malehealthcenter.com
Affiliation: The Male Health Center was founded in 1989 by Dr. Kenneth A. Goldberg, a board-certified urologist. Dr. Goldberg created the center to provide men with an integrated system of care that addressed all their needs.
Mission: To provide information related to male genital health, birth control from the male perspective, and sexual function.
Programs: The Male Health Center was the first center in the United States specializing in male health. It is located in Dallas, Texas, and attracts hundreds of patients from across the United States.

National Campaign to Prevent Teen and Unplanned Pregnancy, The
URL: http://www.thenationalcampaign.org
Phone: (202) 478-8500
Fax: (202) 478-8588
Address: 1776 Massachusetts Avenue, NW
  Suite 200
  Washington, DC 20036
See email form at Web site "Contact Us" section
Affiliation: The National Campaign to Prevent Teen and Unplanned Pregnancy is a nonprofit, nonpartisan organization supported almost entirely by private donations.
Mission: The campaign's mission is to improve the well-being of children, youths, and families by reducing teen pregnancy.

National Herpes Hotline
Phone: (919) 361-8488
Affiliation: The National Herpes Hotline is operated by the American Social Health Association (ASHA) as part of the Herpes Resource Center. The hotline, which receives over 60,000 calls a year, provides accurate information and appropriate referrals to anyone concerned about herpes. Trained health communication specialists are available to address questions related to transmission, prevention, and treatment of herpes simplex virus 1-HSV. The hotline also provides support for emotional issues surrounding herpes, such as self-esteem and partner communication. The hotline is open from 9 A.M. to 6 P.M., ET, Monday through Friday.

National Women's Information Center
URL: http://www.4women.gov
Affiliation: This center is sponsored by the Office on Women's Health of the U.S. Department of Health and Human Services. This Web site serves as a wide-ranging resource center on women's health issues.

Planned Parenthood Federation of America
URL: http://www.plannedparenthood.org
Affiliation: Nonprofit
Mission: Planned Parenthood believes in the fundamental right of each individual, throughout the world, to manage his or her fertility, regardless of the individual's income, marital status, race, ethnicity, sexual orientation, age, national origin, or residence. We believe that respect and value for diversity in all aspects of

our organization are essential to our well-being. We believe that reproductive self-determination must be voluntary and preserve the individual's right to privacy. We further believe that such self-determination will contribute to an enhancement of the quality of life, strong family relationships, and population stability.

Programs: Planned Parenthood provides comprehensive reproductive and complementary health-care services in settings which preserve and protect the essential privacy and rights of each individual; advocates public policies which guarantee these rights and ensure access to such services; provides educational programs which enhance understanding of individual and societal implications of human sexuality; and promotes research and the advancement of technology in reproductive health care and encourages understanding of their inherent bioethical, behavioral, and social implications.

RAINN: Rape, Abuse and Incest National Network

URL: http://www.rainn.org

Phone: (800) 656-HOPE

E-mail: info@rainn.org

Affiliation: RAINN is supported by thousands of individual donors and corporate partners.

Mission: The Rape, Abuse and Incest National Network is the nation's largest anti–sexual assault organization. RAINN operates the National Sexual Assault Hotline at (800) 656-HOPE and carries out programs to prevent sexual assault, help victims, and ensure that rapists are brought to justice.

Programs: With more than 1,000 local affiliates, the National Sexual Assault Hotline has helped more than half a million victims of sexual assault.

Sex Etc.: A Web Page by Teens for Teens

URL: http://www.sxetc.org

Phone: (732) 445-7929

Address: Network for Family Life Education
Center for Applied Psychology
Rutgers University
41 Gordon Road
Suite C
Piscataway, NJ 08854-8067

E-mail: sexetc@rci.rutgers.edu

Affiliation: Sponsored by the Network for Family Life Education, School for Social Work at the Rutgers campus of The State University of New Jersey.

Mission: The mission is to reach millions of teens with positive, balanced, and medically accurate messages about sexual health and to help reduce the high rate of teen pregnancy and sexually transmitted infection in the United States. To reach this goal, they write stories for their Web site and national newsletter, and partner with other national youth media.

Programs: Sex, Etc. is the major component of the National Teen-to-Teen Sexuality Education Project developed by the Network for Family Life Education, a nonprofit organization that provides resources, advocacy, training, and technical assistance in support of balanced, comprehensive sexuality education in the United States. The network is based at the Center for Applied Psychology at the Rutgers campus of the State University of New Jersey.

SIECUS: Sexuality Information and Education Council of the United States

URL: http://www.siecus.org

Phone: (212) 819-9776

Fax: (212) 819-9776

Address: 90 John Street

Suite 704

New York, NY 10038

E-mail: pmalone@siecus.org

Affiliation: SIECUS is a 38-year-old nonprofit organization.

Mission: The Sexuality Information and Education Council of the U.S. is a national, nonprofit organization which affirms that sexuality is a natural and healthy part of living. Incorporated in 1964, SIECUS develops, collects, and disseminates information, promotes comprehensive education about sexuality, and advocates the right of individuals to make responsible sexual choices.

GLOSSARY

abortion the termination of a pregnancy, either spontaneously or by induction

abstinence the practice of not having sex

acquaintance rape sexual assaults committed by someone the victim knows; also known as date rape

adolescence the stage of growth and development between childhood and adulthood entailing major physical, cognitive, emotional, and social changes

AIDS (acquired immunodeficiency syndrome) a chronic disease caused by the human immunodeficiency virus (HIV) in which the immune system is weakened and unable to fight infections

adultery voluntary sexual intercourse between a married person and an individual who is not his or her spouse

amniotic fluid the fluid inside the amniotic sac surrounding the fetus during pregnancy

amniotic sac a thin protective membrane filled with fluid that protects the developing fetus

anal intercourse insertion of a man's penis into the anus of his partner

analingus   oral stimulation, or licking, of the anal regions; also called rimming

anatomy   the structure of the body and the relation of its parts to each other

androgens   a class of hormones that promote physical maturation in males and therefore occur in much higher levels in males than in females.

androgynous   having both male and female characteristics

anesthesia   total or partial loss of feeling or sensation as a result of medications or gases

anonymous testing   testing in which the person who is being tested is not linked by name with the results of his or her test

anorgasmia   the inability to reach orgasm

antiabortion activist   an individual who takes a strong stand against abortion, sometimes by violating the rights of others

antibodies   specialized proteins that fight infection in the body

aphrodisiacs   substances that are believed to arouse sexual desire or increase a person's capacity for sexual activities

autoerotic behaviors   fantasies or erotic dreams

baby blues   a period of sadness and emotional upset due to changing levels of hormones after having a baby; usually lasts a few days

bacterial STDs   sexually transmitted diseases, such as chlamydia, gonorrhea, and syphilis, that are caused by bacteria

barrier methods   contraceptives, such as condoms and the diaphragm, that block the sperm from meeting the egg

birth control pill   a pill that is taken orally to prevent ovulation; part of a hormonal method of birth control

bisexual   emotional and sexual attraction to both males and females

blastocyst   the stage of development from the time a fertilized egg implants itself in the uterus to day 14

blood cholesterol levels   the amount of cholesterol in the blood

body temperature method   a fertility awareness method that determines ovulation by keeping a close record of a woman's body temperature, which usually drops slightly prior to ovulation

Braxton-Hicks   uterine contractions that occur in preparation for labor

breast-feeding   feeding a baby milk from a mother's breast

celibacy   the practice of remaining abstinent

cerebral cortex   the part of the brain that produces fantasies and is responsible for language, imagination, and reasoning; also referred to as the thinking center

cervical cap   a contraceptive method involving a rubber barrier that fits snugly over the cervix to block semen

cervical ectropion   also called cervical erosion, a condition in which the cells from inside the cervix grow on the outside, producing an area of redness; it is not cancerous and does not affect fertility

cervical mucus   naturally occurring mucus secreted by the cervix

cervix   a small opening to the uterus

cesarean section   a surgical procedure in which a physician makes an incision through the abdominal wall and uterus to deliver a baby

child pornography   an image, video, or other form of pornography that involves children

child sexual abuse   contact between a child and an adult in which the child is being used for sexual stimulation of the adult or when the perpetrator is in a position of power or control over the victim

chlamydia   a sexually transmitted disease caused by a bacteria

cholesterol   a necessary, waxy fatlike substance in animal tissue

chromosomes   organized structures of DNA and proteins that are found in cells

circumcision   a surgical procedure in which the foreskin is removed from the penis

civil union   a voluntary union for life (or until divorce) of two adults of the same sex

clitoris   the female organ that serves as the center for sexual arousal, located above the urethral opening

colostrum   yellowish or clear liquid secreted from the breasts that contains antibodies and protein

coming out   openly expressing one's (usually same-sex) sexual orientation

companionate love   love characterized by friendly affection with deep attachment

complete celibacy   the practice of not engaging in any sexual activity, including masturbation

condom   a thin, rubberlike material that covers the penis during sexual intercourse or oral sex to prevent an unwanted pregnancy and/or protect against sexually transmitted diseases

confidential testing   a testing procedure in which the person being tested has his or her name linked with the result of the test, but the information is kept confidential

consummate love   love characterized by passion, intimacy, and commitment

contraceptive patch a one-inch square that is placed on the body to prevent pregnancy by releasing a dose of estrogen and progesterone similar to the dose in a week's supply of birth control pills

contraceptives products used to prevent pregnancy

contractions tightening of the uterus muscle to help push the baby out during labor and delivery

Cowper's glands two male glands located at the side of the urethra that produce pre-ejaculatory fluid

cross-dressing wearing the clothing of a member of the other sex for sexual gratification

culture the way a group of people live; includes attitudes and values

cunnilingus oral sex performed on a woman

curette a metal instrument that scrapes the uterine walls during an abortion

cybersex sexual arousal as a result of images or words on a computer

date rape *See* acquaintance rape.

date rape drugs substances used to facilitate sexual assault by incapacitating the victim with the intent of reducing consciousness, memory, and ability to properly function

dental dam a square piece of latex, similar to a condom, that is placed over the entire female genital area to protect against sexually transmitted diseases during oral sex

Depo-Provera an injection of progesterone given every three months to prevent pregnancy

depressant a drug that slows certain functions of the brain, including the central nervous system, which controls breathing and heart rate

desire the first phase in the sexual response cycle, characterized by an interest in sexual activity or intercourse

diabetes   a condition that occurs when the body cannot regulate the level of sugar in the blood, resulting in deficient insulin and excess sugar in urine and blood

diaphragm   a contraceptive method involving a dome–shaped rubber cap with a flexible rim placed deep inside the vagina to cover the cervix and collect semen

dilation and evacuation   an abortion procedure in which the uterine wall is scraped followed by suctioning to remove the contents of the uterus; also known as a D&E

double standard   the term used to describe an action that is acceptable for one gender but not the other

drug-facilitated rape   a rape involving the use of a date rape drug

dyspareunia   pain during intercourse

ecstasy   an illegal hallucinogenic amphetamine; commonly used as a club drug

ectopic pregnancy   a pregnancy in which the fertilized egg implants in a fallopian tube instead of the uterus

ejaculation   the process of semen being expelled from the body through the penis

elective abortion   ending of a pregnancy before the developing baby is able to survive

embryo   the early form of life in the uterus from week two through week eight

emergency contraception   a high-dose birth control pill given twice within 72 hours of having unprotected sex to prevent pregnancy

empathy   compassion and sympathy

empty love   a relationship in which a couple stays together because both partners feel they have to

epididymis   the comma-shaped organ that lies along the back of each testis; carries sperm to the vas deferens

erogenous zone   a place on the body that has many nerve endings and is therefore highly sensitive

erotic dreams   sexually exciting dreams that occur without conscious control

estrogen   a female hormone produced by the ovaries that is responsible for secondary sexual characteristics in females and for the preparation of the uterus for implantation of the fertilized egg

excitement   the second phase in the sexual response cycle characterized by feelings of arousal, including an increase in heartbeat, pulse, blood pressure, breathing, and blood being sent to the genital area

exhibitionism   the illegal exposure of one's genitals to other people without their consent for sexual gratification

fallopian tubes   two tubes that conduct the egg from the ovary to the uterus; part of the female reproductive system

fantasies   thoughts or daydreams that sexually excite someone

fatuous love   love characterized by passion, but lacking in closeness

fellatio   oral sex performed on a man

fertility   the ability to produce healthy eggs and sperm for reproduction

fertility awareness method   a practice that helps a woman know which days of the month she is most likely to get pregnant by observing her body and charting physical changes

fertilization   the fusion of the mother's egg and the father's sperm

fetal alcohol syndrome   a combination of birth defects caused by the mother's consumption of alcohol during pregnancy.

fetish   excessive or irrational devotion to an object or body that causes sexual arousal

fetus   the unborn child from the second month of pregnancy until birth

folic acid   a nutrient that aids in healthy cell development and strengthens the immune system

foreplay   activity that contributes to sexual excitement

foreskin   the skin that covers the end of the penis

fraternal twins   twins that are the result of two separate eggs being released and fertilized

friendship   a relationship that places importance on sharing closeness and trust

gay   a man who is attracted to another man; a male homosexual

gender   one's femininity or masculinity based on psychological and social characteristics

gender reassignment surgery   surgery to reconstruct one's anatomy to match that of the opposite sex

gender role   a culturally expected pattern of behavior and attitudes determined by whether a person is male or female

genes   biological units of heredity

genital warts   a sexually transmitted disease caused by the human papilloma virus, characterized by painless pink or gray warts around the genital area

GHB (gamma-hydroxybutyrate) an illegal depressant that is a colorless and odorless liquid commonly used to facilitate sexual assault

glans the tip of the penis

glucose a sugar molecule resulting from the breakdown of carbohydrates in the body; a main source of energy, which needs sufficient insulin to leave the blood to be changed into energy

gonadotropins hormones that stimulate the gonads, testes, and ovaries to release more hormones than necessary for reproductive development

gonads the male and female sex glands

gonorrhea a sexually transmitted disease caused by a bacterium

group date a date with several couples

group sex sexual activities between three or more people

herpes a viral sexually transmitted disease causing small, painful, red bumps that become filled with fluid and appear as blisters that will rupture to form wet, open sores

heterosexual emotional and sexual attraction to people of the opposite sex

HIV (human immunodeficiency virus) the virus that causes AIDS

homophobia intense, irrational fear and hatred of homosexuals

homosexual emotional and sexual attraction to people of one's own sex

hormonal method the use of contraceptives, such as birth control pills, to prevent ovulation

hormones   chemical substances that act as messengers within the body to regulate various functions

human chorionic gonadotropin   a hormone released from the time a fertilized egg implants in the uterus through the end of pregnancy

HPV (human papilloma virus)   a group of viruses that include more than 100 different strains, with over 30 infecting the genital area

hyperglycemia   a condition in which a person has too much sugar in his or her blood

hypoglycemia   a condition in which a person has too little sugar in his or her blood

hypothalamus   a part of the brain that regulates body temperature, hunger, feelings of rage, aggressions, pain, pleasure, and patterns of sexual arousal

identical twins   twins that result from a fertilized egg splitting into two

immune system   a system of the body that fights infection

impotence   the inability to achieve and maintain an erection

incest   sexual intercourse between people too closely related to marry

infant mortality   the death of a baby before the child's first birthday

infatuation   love in which one person is completely absorbed with desire for another

infertility   the inability to get pregnant

intercourse   penetration of the penis into the vagina or anus

in the closet a term used to describe a person who chooses not to declare his or her sexual preference

intimacy commitment, caring, and self-disclosure

iron a mineral needed for energy production and growth, found in eggs, fish, meat, green leafy vegetables, and whole grains

labia folds of skin located on each side of the vagina

labia majora the outer lips of the female vulva

labia minora the inner lips of the female vulva

laparoscopy a surgical procedure in which a thin, flexible tube with a lighted end is inserted through a small incision in the lower abdomen

late term abortions abortions performed during the third trimester

lesbian a woman who is attracted to other women; a female homosexual

lightening the lowering of the fetus in the uterus in preparation for birth

limbic system a complex part of the brain comprised of deep nuclei and fiber tracts related to the control and expression of the emotions

low-birth-weight the term used to describe a baby who weighs less than 5.5 pounds at birth

lubricant a water-based jelly or cream to lubricate or moisten the vagina or anus to ease insertion of the penis

Lunelle a monthly contraceptive injection of estrogen and progesterone

macrosomia   a "fat" baby; a condition caused by untreated diabetes in the mother, resulting in health problems in the child

masturbation   stimulation of the genitals with the hands

Medicaid   a federal and state health insurance program designed to provide access to health services for people below a certain income level

menarche   the onset of menstruation

menopause   the end of menstruation due to hormonal changes, surgery or drug use

menstrual cycle   a recurring cycle beginning at menarche and ending at menopause in which the lining of the uterus prepares for possible pregnancy

menstruation   the loss of blood and tissue lining the uterus each month a woman does not become pregnant

minipill   birth control pill that contains only progesterone

miscarriage   spontaneous delivery of a fetus before it is able to live on its own due to complications with the pregnancy

mons vereris   the fatty tissue covering the female pubic bone

morning sickness   feelings of nausea and vomiting early in pregnancy

mucus method   a contraceptive method to determine ovulation by examining changes in the naturally occurring cervical mucus

mucus plug   tissue and blood which covers the cervix during pregnancy to protect the fetus

multiple orgasms   repeated orgasms

nature   biological factors that affect an individual

nocturnal emission orgasm and ejaculation during sleep; also called nocturnal orgasm or a wet dream

Norplant the contraceptive implant that is inserted under the skin of a woman's arm and releases hormones

nurse midwife a registered nurse with additional training in prenatal care and child delivery

nurture life experiences and psychological factors that affect an individual

ob-gyn (obstetrician/gynecologist) a physician trained and certified in obstetrics (prenatal care and delivery) and gynecology (women's reproductive health)

oral-genital stimulation oral sex, the placing of one's mouth or tongue onto a partner's genitals

oral herpes a type of herpes virus, HSV 1, that causes painful sores or blisters on the mouth; also known as cold sores

orgasm pleasurable rhythmic contractions of muscles in the genital area resulting from sexual arousal

outercourse sexual activity that involves a couple rubbing their bodies against each other with no penetration

ovaries paired female organs that produce ova, or eggs, and female hormones

over-the-counter medicines medications that can be purchased without a prescription

ovulation the release of an egg by a female's ovary; the time when a female is most likely to become pregnant

Pap smear a test to detect cancer on the cervix by swabbing fluid from the cervix

parental consent   approval required by some states from at least one parent prior to performing an abortion on a female under age 18

partial celibacy   the practice of not engaging in sexual activity with another person but allowing self masturbation

pedophile   a molester of children or teens

pelvic inflammatory disease   an infection of the fallopian tubes in which scar tissue may form within the tubes and block the passage of eggs and sperm, leading to infertility

penis   the male organ, made up of nerves, blood vessels, and spongy and fibrous tissue

perineum   the area between the anus and the vaginal opening in females and the anus and testes in males

perpetrator   a person who commits a crime

physiology   the science that deals with the functions of an organism or its parts

placenta   an organ through which the fetus receives nourishment

pornography   creative activity of no literary or artistic value other than to stimulate sexual desire

postpartum depression   a mental disorder characterized by sadness, despair, and discouragement experienced by some women following the birth of a baby

post-traumatic stress disorder (PTSD)   a pattern of symptoms experienced by some individuals after a traumatic event such as sexual assault, including memories of the assault, nightmares, avoidance of thoughts, feelings, and situations related to the assault, difficulty sleeping and concentrating, and irritability

precoital fluid   a fluid released from the penis during arousal and prior to ejaculation to neutralize the male's urethra and lubricate the female's vagina

pre-ejaculatory fluid fluid that exits the penis during intercourse before ejaculation; also called pre-ejaculate or pre-cum

premature a term used to describe infants born before they reach full term, or 36 weeks

premature ejaculation ejaculating too quickly after becoming sexually stimulated and excited

private adoption an adoption arranged between those who wish to adopt a baby and the woman who wants to give up custody of her child

pro-choice the belief that women have the right to decide whether or not to terminate their pregnancy

pro-life the belief that women should not have the right to decide whether or not to terminate their pregnancy

progesterone the female hormone that helps maintain pregnancy and regulate the menstrual cycle

prostaglandin induction an abortion procedure conducted by administering prostaglandins to cause uterine contractions resulting in the expulsion of the fetus from the vagina within 24 hours

prostate gland a walnut-sized gland in males, located at the base of the bladder, that produces about 30 percent of semen

prostitution the offering and exchange of sexual acts for money

puberty a period of rapid physical and emotional changes that usually occurs between the ages of 12 and 20

public display of affection (PDA) when two people show affection, generally kissing or touching, in public

rape sexual penetration against a person's will

refractory period the span of time after having an orgasm in which a person is not physically capable of having another orgasm

resolution the fourth stage of the sexual response cycle, character-ized by the body returning to the unexcited state

respiratory distress syndrome an illness in newborns, caused by immaturity of the lungs, in which the air sacs in the lungs do not have the proper structures to remain open during normal breathing; the leading cause of death in premature infants

reproduction the process of producing offspring

rhythm method a contraceptive method based on abstaining from intercourse during the fertile days of a female's menstrual cycle (the period around ovulation)

Rohypnol an illegal depressant that is a colorless and odorless pill commonly used to facilitate sexual assault

romantic love love characterized by closeness and lust but no commitment

RU–486 a drug used to induce abortion

sadomasochism the expression of sexuality through pain; also known as S and M

scrotum the pouch of skin that holds the testes

secondary sex characteristics physical characteristics other than genitals that distinguish males from females

self-esteem a personal feeling of self-worth

semen the fluid that contains sperm and is discharged at ejaculation through the penis

seminal vesicles two small glands that produce most of the fluid in semen

sex biological maleness or femaleness

sex reassignment the surgical alteration of the appearance of genitals to relieve intense cross-gender feelings

sexual assault the use of force or threat to cause another person to engage in an unwanted sexual act

sexuality the emotional, intellectual, and physical aspects of sexual attraction and expression

sexual offender a person who has criminally assaulted another sexually

sexual orientation a consistent pattern of emotional and sexual attraction based on one's biological sex

sexual performance the ability to perform during intercourse

sexual predator a person who has a habit of seeking out sexual satisfaction at the emotional and physical expense of others

sexual response cycle the pattern of physically responding to sexual stimulation, characterized by four stages

SIDS (sudden infant death syndrome) the sudden death of an apparently healthy infant during sleep

sodomy laws laws banning oral sex and anal sex

sonogram a procedure that uses electromagnetic waves to produce a visual image

sperm the male sex cell necessary for reproduction

spermicide a chemical that kills sperm

spontaneous abortion termination of pregnancy due to natural causes at less than 20 weeks' gestation; a miscarriage

statutory rape   intercourse with a person under the age of consent

STD (sexually transmitted disease)   a disease transmitted by sexual contact

stereotype   a label or judgment about an individual based on the characteristics of a group

sterilization   permanent methods of contraception, such as a tubal ligation for women and vasectomy for men

suction curettage   an abortion procedure involving dilation of the cervix and removal of uterine contents by a small plastic tube attached to a vacuum aspirator

syphilis   a sexually transmitted disease caused by a bacterium

testes   the paired male organs that produce sperm and male hormones

testosterone   a hormone, secreted by the adrenal glands and testes in males, needed for sperm development, growth and development of male reproductive organs, secondary sex characteristics, and body growth

toxemia   a condition associated with the presence of toxic matter in the blood, causing high blood pressure and fluid retention

transgender   crossing of traditional gender lines because of discomfort with traditional gender roles

transsexual   a person whose gender identity does not match his or her biological sex

transvestite   a person who wears clothing of the other sex to become sexually aroused

tubal ligation   the surgery for women in which the fallopian tubes are blocked to prevent fertilization

tubo-ovarian abscess a collection of bacteria, pus, and fluid that occurs in a fallopian tube

ultrasound medical imaging technique to see inside the human body using high-frequency sound waves

umbilical cord the cord that connects the fetus to the placenta by which nutrients, oxygen, and waste products pass between the mother and fetus

urethra the tube through which urine passes from the bladder to outside the body; in males, the urethra also serves as a passageway for sperm

urethral opening the opening of the urethra to the outside of the body, located at the tip of the penis in males and above the vaginal opening in females

uterus a hollow organ where the fetus develops

vagina the passage leading from the external female genitalia to the internal reproductive organs; also known as the birth canal

vaginal birth the delivery of a baby through the vagina

vaginal intercourse insertion of the penis into the vagina

vaginal opening the opening that leads to the vagina; located below the urethral opening

vaginal ring a flexible ring inserted in the vagina close to the cervix to prevent pregnancy by releasing hormones

vaginismus strong involuntary contractions of the pelvic muscles experienced by women, which may result in pain when attempting intercourse

vas deferens long, thin sperm-carrying tubes that begin at each testicle and end at the urethra

vasectomy   a permanent contraception method for men in which the vas deferens are cut and tied

vernix   a waxy, protective substance on the fetus's skin

victim   a person injured by another

viral STD   a sexually transmitted disease, such as herpes, genital warts, hepatitis B, or HIV, that is caused by a virus and cannot be cured with an antibiotic

virgin   a person who has not had sexual intercourse

voyeurism   an illegal act in which a person receives sexual gratification from seeing the genitalia of others or witnessing others' sexual behavior

water breaking   when the amniotic sac ruptures in preparation for birth, and water is expelled

welfare   financial assistance provided by local, state, or federal government to needy individuals or families

withdrawal   the removal of the penis from the vagina prior to ejaculation in an attempt to avoid pregnancy

yeast infections   a common vaginal infection characterized by an overgrowth of a fungus normally found in the vagina which can cause itching, redness, and a white discharge

zygote   the first cell that forms after conception

INDEX

Boldface page numbers indicate extensive treatment of a topic.